Did y

- It takes approximate_____ _____ _____ _____ _____ ____ _ full-term baby? And that you'll need to eat an extra 300 calories a day during the second and third trimester of pregnancy?

- As much as 250 milligrams of calcium a day are shuttled through the placenta from your body to your baby's?

- Liquids can aggravate morning sickness?

- Women who fast, even for a period as short as one day, increase their risk of premature labor and delivery?

- Blueberries, raisins and baked beans are three excellent sources of iron?

- There are seven things you should *avoid* eating during pregnancy?

You'll discover everything you need to know about calories, protein, calcium, vitamins, iron, fats, sugar, salt, caffeine, and much more in . . .

THE
PREGNANCY NUTRITION
COUNTER

Annette B. Natow, Ph.D., R.D., and Jo-Ann Heslin, M.A., R.D., are the authors of twelve books on nutrition, including *No-Nonsense Nutrition for Your Baby's First Year*, available from Prentice-Hall. Both are former faculty members of Adelphi University and State University of New York, Downstate Medical Center. They are editors of a nutrition research journal and serve on the editorial advisory boards of *American Baby* and *Environmental Nutrition Newsletter*. They have contributed to *Childbirth Educator*, *Working Mother*, *Healthy Children*, *Sesame Street Parents Guide*, and *Cooking Light* and have taught prenatal nutrition classes to expectant parents for over fifteen years.

Books by Annette B. Natow and Jo-Ann Heslin

The Cholesterol Counter
The Diabetes Carbohydrate and Calorie Counter
The Fat Attack Plan
The Fat Counter
Megadoses
No-Nonsense Nutrition for Kids
The Pocket Encyclopedia of Nutrition
The Pregnancy Nutrition Counter

Published by POCKET BOOKS

The PREGNANCY NUTRITION COUNTER

**Annette B. Natow, Ph.D., R.D.,
and
Jo-Ann Heslin, M.A., R.D.**

Pregnancy Journal by Laura E. Lefkowitz

POCKET **STAR** BOOKS

New York   London   Toronto   Sydney   Tokyo   Singapore

An *Original* Publication of POCKET BOOKS

A Pocket Star Book published by
POCKET BOOKS, a division of Simon & Schuster Inc.
1230 Avenue of the Americas, New York, NY 10020

ISBN: 0-671-69563-0

First Pocket Books printing October 1992

10 9 8 7 6 5 4 3 2 1

POCKET STAR BOOKS and colophon are registered
trademarks of Simon & Schuster Inc.

Printed in the U.S.A.

To our families, who support us through every project: Harry, Allen, Irene, Sarah, Meryl, Laura, Marty, George, Emily, Steven, Joseph, Kristen, and Karen.

A special thank you to all the pregnant women who have asked us so many questions in the last fifteen years; to Vicki Kalajian for all her help; to our editor, Sally Peters; and to our agent, Nancy Trichter.

Without the tireless cooperation of Steven, *The Pregnancy Nutrition Counter* would never have been completed.

At no time is a diet . . . going to bring as big a return as when given to the mother upon whom an infant is depending for all its sustenance.

Mary Swartz Rose, Ph.D.
Feeding the Family
(Macmillan, 1919)

Contents

Introduction

FEEDING YOUR BABY RIGHT—RIGHT FROM THE START

Every pregnancy, like every child, has a personality all its own. The journey you are about to begin is like no other that you will take in your life. As you go through the physical and emotional experiences of pregnancy, your life will be changed forever.

The Mother's Journal, which introduces each month, shares with you some of the experiences, concerns and feelings that Laura, now a new mother, had during her pregnancy. Consider keeping your own Mother's Journal. It can be a wonderful gift for you to share with your child someday.

You're not going to become a mother in a few months—you already are one. The care and feeding of your infant began at the moment of conception. Though you were not aware of it, you began to "mother" your child at that instant. The two of you are an inseparable pair. How you take care of yourself right now directly affects the development of your baby's brain, heart, lungs, and other vital organs. The best way to take good care of your developing baby is to take care of yourself: eat well, exercise, and get plenty of rest.

THREE PHASES OF PREGNANCY

A normal pregnancy, from ovulation to delivery, averages 265 to 280 days, or approximately nine calendar months. It is divided into three stages, or trimesters.

1

During the first trimester—the first three months—your baby is called an embryo. This is the most critical phase for the development of vital organs. Because cells are dividing rapidly and organs are forming, your baby is vulnerable to physical and environmental factors that may affect you. It is especially important, during these months, to avoid exposure to X rays and contagious diseases and to abstain from drugs and alcohol. During the first trimester your body is creating two vital and amazing structures that ensure the support and nourishment of your developing baby: the amniotic sac and the placenta.

Your baby lives and grows enclosed in two sacs. The outer sac is the uterus, and the one surrounding your baby is the amniotic sac or membrane. He floats free in a clear liquid called amniotic fluid, which increases from about 3 ounces at the end of the first trimester to as much as 1½ quarts at term. Water, which makes up 98 percent of the amniotic fluid, is renewed every three hours. Other substances floating in the liquid include proteins and minerals, which are replaced regularly.

The amniotic fluid protects your baby by providing a constant and perfect environment for growth and development. It also functions as a shock absorber so that your daily activities and exercise don't bounce your baby around too much. You replenish the nutrients and remove waste materials from the amniotic fluid through the placenta.

Extending from the wall of your uterus to the baby's umbilical cord, the placenta is the connection or bridge between the two of you. At your end, your blood vessels spiderweb into the placenta and deliver oxygen and nutrients needed for baby's growth, while at the same time picking up carbon dioxide and wastes that need to be removed and excreted. The placental pump sends these substances to and from your baby. His blood vessels spiderweb into the other end of the placenta, picking up those substances needed for development and dropping off wastes.

The placenta is a remarkable structure that has received much attention and study by experts. You can think about it as your baby's life-support system, much like the kind an astronaut uses in space. It filters your baby's blood at the umbilical end, removing wastes and continuously replenishing the baby's supply of oxygen, nutrients, and protein so that growth can proceed uninterrupted.

This available stockpile of nutrients comes from you. The food you take in each day is broken down and absorbed into your bloodstream and delivered at regular intervals to the placental circulation to be ferried across to your baby. Although the placenta is amazing it is not flawless. It is unable, in most cases, to distinguish between needed substances and harmful substances. It recognizes substances simply by the concentration in the mother's blood and pumps a like concentration across to the baby. This means that if you have a high concentration of alcohol, drugs, or nicotine in your blood, the placenta will deliver a like concentration to your baby. It was once believed that this structure was a magical barrier that protected the developing baby from harm, but today we realize that the placenta is simply an efficient delivery system. It is up to you to deliver the "right stuff" to your baby.

The placenta forms during the first few weeks of pregnancy and begins to function around the sixth week. It performs optimally until shortly before delivery. This aging and slowing down may be necessary to trigger labor.

The middle of pregnancy, months 4 to 6, is the second trimester. Your baby is completely formed, but a refinement of organs and body systems is still needed. Now your baby is called a fetus. Though unable to live independently, the fetus is far more developed than the more primitive embryo. She is also bigger and quite active. This is the point in pregnancy where many women swear they are going to give birth to an acrobat!

As your weight creeps up and your belly begins to bulge noticeably, many women start to worry about their weight gain and wonder if they shouldn't cut back on what they are eating. Always remember that the two of you are an inseparable pair, sharing equally in resources. If you eat well, both you and your baby receive needed nutrients. When you skip meals and make poor food choices so does your developing baby. This is not the time to diet or start some unusual eating regimen that might jeopardize your baby's growth. Gaining the appropriate amount of weight is one of the most important things you can do to ensure your baby's future health.

In the last trimester, months seven through nine, nutrient demands are at their greatest as your baby goes through his final growth spurt before birth. Fetal weight triples during this trimester to an average birth weight of about seven pounds. Brain, muscles, bones, and fatty tissues are growing rapidly, and the liver, lungs, adrenal glands, and diaphragm are maturing. To meet baby's increased demands, the absorptive capacity and transport efficiency of the placenta reach a peak in the third trimester and then slowly decline just before birth.

A woman's body undergoes many changes during the nine months of pregnancy. Heart rate increases to circulate the increased amount of blood. The lung capacity increases, and a pregnant woman actually uses 15 percent more oxygen. The renal (kidney) track dilates and holds more urine. The urge to urinate increases in early pregnancy, followed by increased thirst. This is your body's mechanism to replace lost water and provide necessary additional fluids. In addition to your body changes, you are producing your baby's life-support system that will allow the baby to develop over the next nine months.

All of this activity requires extra energy and the building blocks, or raw materials, needed to support the growth of new tissues in your body and in your baby's. Energy can be translated into calories, and you will need extra calories each day. Building blocks of new body tissues are protein and other vital nutrients like iron, calcium, vitamin C, and folic acid (a B vitamin). Each of these serves a unique function that allows your unborn baby to develop into a healthy full-term infant.

"THE RIGHT STUFF"

Your nutritional needs during pregnancy are unique at this time in your life. It has been estimated that it takes approximately 55,000 calories to support the growth of a full-term baby. This translates into 300 extra calories a day during the second and third trimester. Because your baby is so small and requires so little energy for development during the first trimester, experts now agree that pregnant women do not need extra calories during this period.

Protein is required to form all new cells. By the time your baby is born, 925 grams of protein will have gone into the cells of his body and into the extra tissue that has been produced in various parts of your body, like the breasts, uterus, and placenta. Calculated over an entire pregnancy, you will need 10 extra grams of protein a day.

Vitamin C is the "cementing agent" that holds new cells together. It helps to form your baby's connective tissue, skin, and tendons. An additional 10 milligrams a day will easily meet this increased need.

The need for folic acid, a B vitamin, more than doubles during pregnancy. This makes sense when you realize that this vitamin is involved in the process of normal cell division. At birth your new baby will be a bundle of billions of cells that were formed over the nine months of pregnancy.

The need for iron is high to enable you and your baby to form new red blood cells. These cells are responsible for carrying oxygen in the body and allowing you to deliver the necessary oxygen to the placenta for your baby. Not only is your baby producing new red blood cells but a supply of iron is being stored away in baby's body for use in early infancy. At birth a normal-weight infant has about 246 milligrams of iron in his blood and body stores. An additional 134 milligrams of iron are stored in the placenta and about 290 milligrams of iron have been used in the expansion of your blood supply.

Meeting adequate iron needs throughout pregnancy is a challenge, since it is estimated that the average American diet supplies approximately 6 milligrams of iron per 1,000 calories eaten. It is recommended that pregnant women get 30 milligrams of iron daily, throughout pregnancy. Because many women enter pregnancy with less than adequate iron stores, many doctors routinely recommend an iron supplement to their patients. If your doctor does this, it is still important for you to eat good food sources of iron, since the absorption of iron is greater from food than from supplements.

Calcium is important during pregnancy to ensure the development of bones and teeth. Your baby will need the most calcium in the last trimester when bones are hardening. It has been estimated that 13 milligrams of calcium an hour, or 250 to 300 milligrams a day, are shuttled through the placenta to your baby. By birth your baby's body will have accumulated approximately 25 grams (25,000 milligrams) of calcium. To maintain the health of your own skeleton and to help build your baby's skeleton, experts recommend that you get 1,200 milligrams of calcium each day throughout your pregnancy.

Energy (calories), protein, vitamin C, folic acid, iron, and calcium are "the right stuff"—the key nutrients that help to ensure a successful pregnancy. It is important throughout pregnancy to have adequate amounts of these key nutrients. The table, Nutrient Needs of Women, on page 8, provides a very clear picture of how nutrient demands go up during pregnancy. To meet those demands, you will need to eat a wide variety of healthful foods every day.

TRACKING KEY NUTRIENTS

The Pregnancy Nutrition Counter was designed to help make the job of eating right easier for you. On at least one day during each week of pregnancy write down everything you eat on that day. The Pregnancy Food Checklist was designed as a handy tool to help you do this. A sample of the checklist is provided on pages 10–11. Additional checklists will be found throughout each month of your Pregnancy Counter as a reminder to keep track of the important key nutrients.

Once you have written down everything you have eaten during that one day, use the nutrient counter beginning on page 135 and list the amount of each key nutrient contributed by every food you have eaten. The subtotals and daily total will serve as checks to see how close you are coming to your nutrient goals for the day. On pages 10–11 is a sample checklist. The nutrient goals were met for all the key nutrients except iron.

This is how you should go about checking and, when needed, altering your food intake throughout pregnancy:

1. Record a sample day during each week of pregnancy.
2. Calculate the amount of each key nutrient eaten that day.
3. If you fall short of any of the key nutrients, change your food choices to be sure you've included all the key nutrients you and your developing baby need.

Why not fill out the sample on page 12 right now, to see how the two of you are doing?

MORE ABOUT KEY NUTRIENTS

In this section of *The Pregnancy Nutrition Counter* you have had a brief introduction to the key nutrients and how to track them. No one expects you to change your food habits overnight. Since it takes nine months for your baby to develop, you can use the next nine months to practice making good food choices. Each month one of the key nutrients will be highlighted to help you easily understand its importance to a successful pregnancy.

By learning a little more about nutrition each month, by putting what you learn into practice as you track key nutrients, and by changing your diet to the most healthful food choices, you will be practicing good eating habits that you can use for the rest of your life. By the time your baby is born, good eating practices will have become habits—practices you do so naturally you don't even need to think about them. At this point it will be time to teach these good eating habits to your child. That's why it's so important to feed yourself and your baby right—right from the start.

YOU'LL LEARN MORE ABOUT—

Protein	in Month	1
Folic Acid	in Month	2
Vitamin C	in Month	3
Iron	in Month	4
Calcium	in Month	5

NUTRIENT NEEDS OF WOMEN

Nutrient	Adult	Trimesters			Breast-feeding	
		First	Second	Third	Mo. 1–6	Mo. 7–12
Calories	2,200	no extra need	+300	+300	+500	+500
Protein	50g	60g	60g	60g	65g	62g
Vitamin C	60mg	70mg	70mg	70mg	95mg	90mg
Folic Acid (a B vitamin)	180mcg	400mcg	400mcg	400mcg	280mcg	260mcg
Calcium	800mg[3] 1,200mg[4]	1,200mg	1,200mg	1,200mg	1,200mg	1,200mg
Iron	15mg	30mg	30mg	30mg	15mg	30mg*

1. Based on Recommended Dietary Allowances, 10th edition, 1989, National Academy of Sciences.
2. Nutrient needs reflect average breast milk production of women in the United States. Nutrient needs decrease slightly during second six months of breast-feeding because most babies are now getting some needs from the addition of solid food.
3. Requirement for women age twenty-five and older.
4. Requirement for women age nineteen to twenty-five.
* Getting this much iron through food is a real challenge. A good goal: Try to consume 15mg of iron from food sources and take the iron supplement recommended by your doctor.

8

DAILY FOOD GUIDE TO
KEY NUTRIENTS NEEDED
DURING PREGNANCY

To be sure that you get all the key nutrients you and your developing baby need each day, follow this daily food guide. Each day have:

2 to 3 servings (4 to 6 ounces)	protein-rich foods
4 servings	calcium-rich food
5 servings	fruits and vegetables
5 or more servings	breads, cereals, grains (whole grain and enriched varieties)

TRACKING KEY NUTRIENTS ON THE
PREGNANCY FOOD CHECKLIST

1. Record a sample day during each week of pregnancy.
2. Calculate the amount of each key nutrient eaten that day.
3. If you fall short of any of the key nutrients, change your food choices to be sure you've included all the key nutrients you and your developing baby need.

SAMPLE

PREGNANCY FOOD CHECKLIST

	CAL	PRO (G)	VIT C (MG)	FOL (MCG)	CA (MG)	IR (MG)
BREAKFAST:						
½ cup orange juice	55	1	41	23	12	*tr
⅓ cup All-Bran	70	4	15	—	23	5
1 cup whole milk	150	8	2	12	291	tr
1 slice white bread	65	2	tr	—	32	1
1 pat butter	36	tr	0	tr	1	tr
1 cup tea	2	0	0	9	0	tr
Subtotal	378	15	58	44	359	6
SNACK:						
8 ounces low-fat coffee yogurt	194	11	2	24	389	tr
1 tablespoon wheat germ	27	2	tr	25	7	1
Subtotal	599	28	60	93	755	7
LUNCH:						
Cheese sandwich						
2 slices whole wheat bread	140	6	tr	—	20	1
2 ounces American cheese	212	12	0	4	358	tr
1 tomato, sliced	24	1	22	12	8	1
1 teaspoon mayonnaise	33	tr	—	—	tr	tr
Spinach Salad						
1 cup chopped spinach	12	2	16	108	56	2
¼ cup raw carrot, shredded	12	tr	3	4	8	tr
1 tablespoon Reduced Calorie French dressing	22	0	—	—	2	tr
1 glass club soda	0	0	0	0	17	0
Subtotal	1054	49	101	221	1224	11
SNACK:						
2 shortbread cookies	77	1	0	—	7	tr
1 cup hot cocoa, made with water	103	3	1	tr	96	tr
Subtotal	1234	53	102	221	1327	11

DINNER:

½ cantaloupe	94	2	113	46	28	1
5 ounces chicken, dark meat without skin	286	38	0	11	21	2
1 large (6½ ounce) baked potato with skin	220	5	26	22	20	3
½ cup snap beans, cooked	22	1	6	21	29	1
½ cup applesauce	53	tr	2	1	4	tr
1 cup tea	2	0	0	9	0	tr
Subtotal	1911	99	249	331	1429	18

SNACK:

1 ounce peanuts	164	7	0	41	15	1
1 cup lemonade	100	tr	10	6	8	tr
Subtotal	2175	106	259	378	1452	19
Daily Totals	2175	106	259	378	1452	19
Daily Nutrient Goals	2200	60	70	400	1200	15

*tr = trace

PREGNANCY FOOD CHECKLIST						
	CAL	PRO (G)	VIT C (MG)	FOL (MCG)	CA (MG)	IR (MG)
BREAKFAST:						
Subtotal	——	——	——	——	——	——
SNACK:						
Subtotal	——	——	——	——	——	——
LUNCH:						
Subtotal	——	——	——	——	——	——
SNACK:						
Subtotal	——	——	——	——	——	——
DINNER:						
Subtotal	——	——	——	——	——	——
SNACK:						
Subtotal	——	——	——	——	——	——
Daily Totals	——	——	——	——	——	——
Daily Nutrient Goals	2200	60	70	400	1200	30

THE

FIRST

TRIMESTER

MONTH 1

A Mother's Journal

WEEK 1

WEEK 2

WEEK 3

WEEK 4

During the last month I have been noticing some changes in my body: my breasts have been tender and achy, I've been belching after most meals and snacks, and I'm urinating so frequently that I'm planning my days so I'm not far from a toilet. Three times this week, while preparing dinner, my face became hot and sweaty. Now I know what a hot flash is!

YOUR BABY

From a single microscopic fertilized egg, your baby develops into a ¼-inch embryo. Though this may seem incredibly tiny to you, by the end of the first month, your baby will be 10,000 times larger than at conception. Heart, brain, spinal cord, and digestive tract begin to form. Before the end of the month, your baby's heart will be beating.

YOUR BODY

Your period is now about two weeks late, and you are approximately one month pregnant. If you are like most women, this first month, for the most part, passed before you even realized you were pregnant.

Though you've been unaware of it, the magic of your pregnancy has already begun. Your baby's development began at fertilization, when a sperm and an ovum (egg) united to form a single-cell organism called a zygote; 22,896,000 seconds after this happens your baby will be born. Through growth and cell division the zygote develops into an embryo.

While all this is happening, your body may be giving off signals that something is up. Your breasts may feel tender and full, similar to the way they usually feel before a period, but now the tenderness remains. You may be feeling queasy in the morning and find you have to urinate very frequently. You also may feel blue and find that otherwise normal tastes and smells are now peculiar.

So this is pregnancy!

FIRST SIGNS OF PREGNANCY:

Missed period

Breast tenderness

Unexplainable fatigue

Sensitivity to strong odors

Metallic taste in the mouth

Slight rise in body temperature—about 1°

Increased vaginal discharge

Frequent urination

MORNING SICKNESS

Your alarm rings. You shut it off and jump out of bed. Out of nowhere an all-consuming wave of nausea overwhelms you, and the next thing you know you are in the bathroom throwing up. Fifty percent of all pregnant women experience morning sickness. That's the bad news. The good news is that, for almost everyone, it's gone by the end of the third month.

The best way to handle morning sickness is not to let it get started. First, no more jumping out of bed the minute the alarm goes off. Sudden movements, like getting out of bed too quickly, seem to trigger the nausea that can lead to morning vomiting. Set your alarm for a few minutes earlier. Starting right now, morning is going to become a more leisurely affair.

Even though food may be the last thing on your mind when you feel nauseated, during pregnancy, eating will make the sensation subside. At night, before you go to bed, place three or four dry crackers on your night table. As soon as you get up in the morning—before your lift your head off the pillow—eat the crackers slowly and rest, lying down quietly, for another five minutes. Now get up slowly and start the day.

Most women feel better as the day goes on; others may be bothered with queasiness later in the morning or throughout the day. Vomiting, other than in the morning, is rare. If your nausea persists into the day, you may be able to tolerate small frequent meals better than three large meals a day. Skipping meals or going for long periods without food often causes more queasiness. Keep food handy, in your pocketbook or desk, all the time.

Carbohydrate foods—bread, crackers, unbuttered popcorn, cereal, toast, and baked potatoes—go down easily and calm your unsettled stomach. So do hard-cooked eggs. Remember—eating helps, so don't be afraid to eat, thinking things will get worse. They won't.

Liquids, on the other hand, can aggravate nausea. A first course of soup can trigger nausea and ruin the meal. Sipping beverages in between meals is a better idea. Apple juice, grape juice, ginger ale, and cola can all be soothing. Filling up on soda is never a good idea, but a cola or two a day, for the time being, is fine, especially if it makes you feel better and allows you to eat regular meals.

Some women find that a particular food may trigger their nausea. Sometimes it is the odor of the food that is annoying. Brewing coffee, frying fish, and cooking cauliflower are often noted as troublesome. If that happens to you, simply eliminate the food from your diet for the time being.

Though morning sickness can be a real drag, many experts believe that it is a positive sign that your body is going through the necessary hormonal changes needed to support a healthy pregnancy. As a matter of fact, women who have morning sickenss statistically have fewer complications later on.

YOUR DIET: PROTEIN

Billions of tiny cells need to be produced to transform your baby from a microscopic embryo to a full-term healthy baby. Protein-rich foods provide the building material needed to make your baby's body and to keep your body cells in good repair. Additionally you are growing, too—breast tissue, uterine tissue, the placenta, and new blood cells. All of this maintenance, building, and repair requires extra protein.

The Food and Nutrition Board of the National Academy of Sciences recommends that pregnant women get 60 grams of protein a day. This daily amount meets the need to replace worn-out maternal cells; allows for normal growth of the developing baby; lets new maternal tissues, like the uterus, grow; and lets your body store adequate protein.

Translated into food, this means you should be eating 6 to 8 ounces of protein a day. An easy way to estimate 8 ounces is by remembering that a piece of boneless meat, fish, or poultry the size of your palm and as thick as the spot where your little finger joins your palm will weigh about 4 ounces. Eating twice this amount each day guarantees you will meet your extra need for protein throughout pregnancy. Many other foods provide protein as well. The list, "Protein Power," on page 20 will give you some alternatives to meat, fish, and poultry.

Eight percent of your total weight gain during pregnancy is protein. Of that portion, 60 percent is distributed in your baby's body. The baby receives a continuous supply of protein from you via the placenta. The protein foods you eat are broken down into protein fragments called amino acids. The amino acids are delivered to your baby, who reassembles them into whatever organ or body part is under construction at that time.

Early in pregnancy, your tissues—breast, uterus, placenta, and blood—are growing faster than your baby's body. But the reverse will soon be true. By the last trimester, your baby will need practically all the extra protein to complete his growth before birth.

Pregnant women in the United States almost always eat adequate amounts of protein. You really don't need to worry too much about getting enough but you should think about the type of protein foods you choose. Select a good source of protein at each meal and stick with lean choices. This means a pork roast or pork chop rather than sausage or spareribs, skinless chicken rather than duck, and lean ground beef rather than ground chuck. Eat low-fat cheese and substitute beans or tofu in place of meat on occasion. Most people are cautious of too many eggs nowadays, assuming they are high in cholesterol. A medium egg does have 213 milligrams of cholesterol, but it also has only 80 calories and is an excellent source of protein. The cholesterol is found in the egg yolk, the protein is mainly in the egg white. Next time you make scrambled eggs, discard one yolk and scramble the remaining white and one whole egg. Now you have all the protein but only half the cholesterol found in a two-egg portion. (For more information on cholesterol see Month 8.)

Go easy! It's very easy to meet your extra protein needs through food during pregnancy. Protein powders and high-protein drinks are not necessary and may not be the best source of protein for you and your developing baby.

PROTEIN POWER

All of the following choices have the same amount of protein as 2 ounces of meat, fish, or poultry:

- 2 eggs
- 2 ounces cheese
- ½ cup cottage cheese
- ½ cup ricotta cheese
- 1 cup cooked dried beans, any variety
- 1 cup cooked lentils
- 2 to 3 ounces nuts*
- 4 tablespoons of peanut butter*
- 2 ounces pumpkin or sunflower seeds*
- 6 ounces tofu

*These choices are high in fat, use them occasionally.

GIVE SOME THOUGHT TO ALCOHOL

Experts agree that drinking large amounts of alcohol during pregnancy will cause severe damage to your developing baby. The question no one can answer is "How much is too much?" In a large study done by the National Institutes of Health, only one or two drinks a day significantly increased the risk for lower birth weight, which in turn increases the baby's risk for other health problems.

Alcohol crosses the placenta freely, and the alcohol content of the baby's blood will be the same as the mother's. The problem is that the baby's immature liver is unable to break down the alcohol as efficiently as the mother's liver can. This results in a potentially damaging substance circulating through baby's delicate developing body for twice as long as the alcohol would normally stay in the mother's body.

The best advice: *Don't drink at all during pregnancy.*

DAILY FOOD GUIDE TO
KEY NUTRIENTS NEEDED
DURING PREGNANCY

To be sure that you get all the key nutrients you and your developing baby need each day, follow this daily food guide. Each day have:

2 to 3 servings (4 to 6 ounces)	protein-rich foods
4 servings	calcium-rich food
5 servings	fruits and vegetables
5 or more servings	breads, cereals, grains (whole grain and enriched varieties)

TRACKING KEY NUTRIENTS ON THE
PREGNANCY FOOD CHECKLIST

1. Record a sample day during each week of pregnancy.
2. Calculate the amount of each key nutrient eaten that day.
3. If you fall short of any of the key nutrients, change your food choices to be sure you've included all the key nutrients you and your developing baby need.

PREGNANCY FOOD CHECKLIST
Month 1

	CAL	PRO (G)	VIT C (MG)	FOL (MCG)	CA (MG)	IR (MG)
BREAKFAST:						
Subtotal	—	—	—	—	—	—
SNACK:						
Subtotal	—	—	—	—	—	—
LUNCH:						
Subtotal	—	—	—	—	—	—
SNACK:						
Subtotal	—	—	—	—	—	—
DINNER:						
Subtotal	—	—	—	—	—	—
SNACK:						
Subtotal	—	—	—	—	—	—
Daily Totals	—	—	—	—	—	—
Daily Nutrient Goals	2200	60	70	400	1200	30

<u>MONTH 1</u>

Month _____ Year _____

Your feelings:
_____
_____
_____
_____
_____
_____

Your questions for your doctor or nurse-midwife:
_____
_____
_____
_____
_____
_____
_____
_____
_____
_____

MONTH 2

A Mother's Journal

WEEK 5

WEEK 6

WEEK 7

Early this morning, after testing my urine with a home pregnancy detection kit, sure enough, a dark circle appeared, indicating a positive result for pregnancy. We both took a second and even a third long stare into the test tube to convince ourselves that this was real. While I was getting dressed for work I wondered how valid this test was. I couldn't believe that a baby was developing inside me! According to my calculations, I'm already seven weeks pregnant.

WEEK 8

All week I have been thinking about our baby and I'm getting a little anxious about the pregnancy. I'm excited and happy, but I'm also nervous and feel extremely unprepared. My knowledge of infants is slim, and the responsibility seems overwhelming. I now understand why it takes nine months for a baby to fully develop, because it takes about that much time for a mother to prepare herself! I've purchased a few books. Maybe they will help.

YOUR BABY

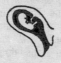

At two months your baby has developed sufficiently to be called a fetus. She is about 1½ inches long, her arms and legs are "budding," and her face is forming eyes, nose, lips, and a tongue. All the major internal organs have formed and are rapidly developing. Though you are unaware of it, your baby is already moving around inside you.

YOUR BODY

At some point during this second month you will make your first visit to the doctor, who will confirm what you already know: you are pregnant!

You've probably already noticed that your weight is beginning to creep up. Weight gains of one-half pound to four pounds are average for the second month. The placenta has begun functioning and is making regular deliveries of vital nutrients to your baby. It is also producing progesterone, the pregnancy-maintaining hormone. This hormone stimulates growth, and most likely you'll soon be needing a larger bra size. Your hair may seem fuller and thicker, too. And your face may become oilier, causing a noticeable change in your complexion. Some women develop clearer skin while others have a bout with blemishes. Your uterus is growing, too—it is now about the size of an egg—but its growth is not yet obvious to you. As the uterus continues to grow, it puts pressure on your bladder and bowel.

BATHROOM BOTHERS

The beginning and end of pregnancy are often marked by the amount of time you spend in the bathroom. Position means a lot in life, and it is the unfortunate position of your bladder to lie between your uterus and your pubic bone. This results in reduced capacity to hold fluids, which sends you to the bathroom every ten minutes! This annoyance will pass shortly, only to return again just before delivery when your baby's head drops into position for birth.

Constipation can also be a bother early in pregnancy. It is important to let your doctor know if you are constipated. Do not take any medications or an enema without your doctor's advice. For some, this temporary problem is just a result of the natural slowing-down of the digestive tract that occurs during pregnancy. You can solve this problem by eating foods that are high in fiber, drinking plenty of fluids, taking a nice long walk each day, and not ignoring the urge to pass a bowel movement. For others, constipation is a signal that the uterus is inverted (tipped the wrong way). The doctor can remedy this problem easily by manipulating the position of the uterus until your baby gets large and heavy enough to keep the uterus in the right position. That is why it is important to tell your doctor if you are constipated.

For more advice on handling constipation see Month 7, where the problem often comes up again.

Your Due Date

Pregnancy, the time from ovulation to delivery, averages 265 to 280 days. To figure out your expected due date, add seven days to the first day of your last menstrual period and count back three months.

This is an approximate date of delivery. Only one in twenty women delivers on her due date. Most deliver sometime within two weeks on either side of this guesstimated date.

My due date is _____

A WORD ABOUT TESTS

Today many tests are available to monitor the health of your developing baby. If you have seen your doctor for a preconception visit you may have already had blood and urine tests. If not, you will have them during your first visit. The results of these tests are another way your doctor monitors your health and that of your baby during pregnancy.

During your first prenatal visit you will have a blood test to determine your blood type and the presence or absence of the RH blood factor. Your blood will also be checked for anemia, because pregnant women are more susceptible to iron-deficiency anemia. Most physicians repeat this test after the fourth month of pregnancy when your developing baby's iron needs increase and your stores of this mineral may become depleted.

Your urine will be checked for bacteria, protein, and sugar at every prenatal visit. These tests may signal a urinary tract infection that can be treated with antibiotics, or they may indicate the need for further testing to see if you are handling sugar normally.

Chorionic villi sampling (CVS) is generally recommended for women who are age forty or older. A sample is taken from the membrane around the baby. This test can be done early in pregnancy, during the second month, and can detect many of the same problems as amniocentesis, which is not done until later on. CVS is done if your doctor feels that you may be at risk and wants to see how your baby is developing.

YOUR DIET: FOLIC ACID

Vitamins act like the body's spark plugs, setting off an endless number of processes necessary to life. Folic acid, a B vitamin, helps to form red and white blood cells and the genetic material inside every cell in the body. Since your baby will be producing billions of cells over the next nine months, it is obvious that this is a very important vitamin during pregnancy.

The Food and Nutrition Board of the National Academy of Sciences recommends that pregnant women get 400 micrograms (mcg) of folic acid a day. This is more than double the 180 micrograms recommended for adult women. In the past it was common for pregnant women to take a folic acid supplement. Many doctors still recommend this to their patients. Experts, however, feel that the current recommended level can be met through food. They no longer recommend routine supplementation for all pregnant women.

A supplement of 300 micrograms a day is recommended in certain situations. Women who used oral contraceptives for a long time before they became pregnant may have lower than normal levels of folic acid in their body stores. Many experts feel they would benefit from a supplement during pregnancy. Women carrying more than one baby may also find it hard to meet increased needs with food. And some women simply do not eat food sources of folic acid and may need a supplement. If you fall into this last group you would be wise to try to increase the variety of foods you eat, since food is always the best source of any nutrient.

Folic acid is found in many foods. Green leafy vegetables, asparagus, oranges, orange juice, ready-to-eat fortified breakfast cereals, wheat germ, nuts, and dried peas and beans are excellent sources. Many people in the United States fall short in their daily consumption of fruits and vegetables. You should be eating five servings a day, but only 9 percent of all adults eat that many. Pregnancy is a good time to initiate this habit to ensure your future health and to be sure you and your developing baby are getting enough folic acid.

Folic acid can be destroyed during storage, preparation, and cooking. To maintain optimum levels of this important vitamin, store fruits and vegetables in a cool place. Stored on the kitchen counter, fruits and vegetables can lose up to 70 percent of their folic acid content within three days. To prevent vitamin loss while cooking, steam or microwave these foods for the shortest time in the smallest possible amount of water. Chilled raw fruits and vegetables have the greatest amount of the vitamin. Eat raw varieties often. Raw salads with a variety of leafy greens are a very rich source of folic acid. Orange juice is a good source of folic acid. This juice offers other bonuses—necessary fluid and a key nutrient, vitamin C—along with folic acid. Drinking a generous serving of orange juice every day is a good food choice.

EXCELLENT SOURCES OF FOLIC ACID

To meet your increased demand for folic acid throughout pregnancy, eat some of these excellent sources each day:

Asparagus
Brussels sprouts
Broccoli
Collard greens
Romaine lettuce
Spinach
Turnip greens
Orange juice
Oranges

Wheat germ
Ready-to-eat fortified breakfast
   cereal
Pinto beans
Lima beans
Lentils
Peanuts
Cashews

Folic Acid

Folic acid is the most commonly used name for a group of chemically similar compounds. The word is derived from the Latin word *folium*, meaning "leaf," and indeed green leafy vegetables are the most outstanding source of this B vitamin.

On food and vitamin labels folic acid is sometimes called folacin or folate.

WHAT THE RESEARCHERS ARE SAYING:

Recent evidence from a number of studies shows a connection between adequate folic acid intake and the prevention of neural tube defect and spina bifida in newborns. This is another important reason to be sure you get enough of this vital nutrient, especially now, early in pregnancy, when your baby's vital organs are forming.

GIVE SOME THOUGHT TO MEGADOSES

Megadoses are large amounts of vitamins and minerals—ten or more times larger than your daily recommended need. It is almost impossible to take in that much in food, but it is not hard to take large amounts of nutrients in the form of pills or tablets. Contrary to popular belief, there is no pre-sale approval of vitamin and mineral supplements. Existing laws do not allow the Food and Drug Administration to limit the quantity of nutrients in a single pill, with the exception of folic acid. Excesses of one nutrient may create a nutritional imbalance or an increased need for other nutrients. Large amounts of some nutrients can be dangerous to your developing baby.

Most vitamins and minerals are needed by the body in very small amounts. Even though your need for these nutrients increases during pregnancy, the increase is small and can easily be met through food. If your doctor recommends a prenatal vitamin and mineral supplement, the amount provided in this supplement will no more than double your daily recommended level. This is a safe increase, nowhere near a megadose.

The best advice: *If you routinely take large doses of nutrients, discontinue this practice while you are pregnant. Discuss nutrient supplementation with your doctor and follow her advice. Select a wide variety of healthful foods as your best source of nutrients.*

DAILY FOOD GUIDE TO
KEY NUTRIENTS NEEDED
DURING PREGNANCY

To be sure that you get all the key nutrients you and your developing baby need each day, follow this daily food guide. Each day have:

2 to 3 servings (4 to 6 ounces)	protein-rich foods
4 servings	calcium-rich food
5 servings	fruits and vegetables
5 or more servings	breads, cereals, grains (whole grain and enriched varieties)

TRACKING KEY NUTRIENTS ON THE
PREGNANCY FOOD CHECKLIST

1. Record a sample day during each week of pregnancy.
2. Calculate the amount of each key nutrient eaten that day.
3. If you fall short of any of the key nutrients, change your food choices to be sure you've included all the key nutrients you and your developing baby need.

PREGNANCY FOOD CHECKLIST
Month 2, Week 1

	CAL	PRO (G)	VIT C (MG)	FOL (MCG)	CA (MG)	IR (MG)
BREAKFAST:						
Subtotal	—	—	—	—	—	—
SNACK:						
Subtotal	—	—	—	—	—	—
LUNCH:						
Subtotal	—	—	—	—	—	—
SNACK:						
Subtotal	—	—	—	—	—	—
DINNER:						
Subtotal	—	—	—	—	—	—
SNACK:						
Subtotal	—	—	—	—	—	—
Daily Totals	—	—	—	—	—	—
Daily Nutrient Goals	2200	60	70	400	1200	30

PREGNANCY FOOD CHECKLIST
Month 2 Week 2

	CAL	PRO (G)	VIT C (MG)	FOL (MCG)	CA (MG)	IR (MG)
BREAKFAST:						
Subtotal	___	___	___	___	___	___
SNACK:						
Subtotal	___	___	___	___	___	___
LUNCH:						
Subtotal	___	___	___	___	___	___
SNACK:						
Subtotal	___	___	___	___	___	___
DINNER:						
Subtotal	___	___	___	___	___	___
SNACK:						
Subtotal	___	___	___	___	___	___
Daily Totals	___	___	___	___	___	___
Daily Nutrient Goals	2200	60	70	400	1200	30

PREGNANCY FOOD CHECKLIST
Month 2, Week 3

	CAL	PRO (G)	VIT C (MG)	FOL (MCG)	CA (MG)	IR (MG)
BREAKFAST:						
Subtotal	—	—	—	—	—	—
SNACK:						
Subtotal	—	—	—	—	—	—
LUNCH:						
Subtotal	—	—	—	—	—	—
SNACK:						
Subtotal	—	—	—	—	—	—
DINNER:						
Subtotal	—	—	—	—	—	—
SNACK:						
Subtotal	—	—	—	—	—	—
Daily Totals	—	—	—	—	—	—
Daily Nutrient Goals	2200	60	70	400	1200	30

PREGNANCY FOOD CHECKLIST
Month 2, Week 4

	CAL	PRO (G)	VIT C (MG)	FOL (MCG)	CA (MG)	IR (MG)
BREAKFAST:						
Subtotal	——	——	——	——	——	——
SNACK:						
Subtotal	——	——	——	——	——	——
LUNCH:						
Subtotal	——	——	——	——	——	——
SNACK:						
Subtotal	——	——	——	——	——	——
DINNER:						
Subtotal	——	——	——	——	——	——
SNACK:						
Subtotal	——	——	——	——	——	——
Daily Totals	——	——	——	——	——	——
Daily Nutrient Goals	2200	60	70	400	1200	30

MONTH 2

Month _____   Year _____

Your feelings:

_____

_____

_____

_____

_____

_____

Your questions for your doctor or nurse-midwife:

_____

_____

_____

_____

_____

_____

_____

_____

_____

_____

_____

_____

MONTH 3

A Mother's Journal

WEEK 9

I've been reading the maternity and child care books to the point of nausea—help! I am also being very careful about my diet. I have stopped drinking soda and have reduced the amount of coffee and tea I drink. I'm very tired.

WEEK 10

Today I had my first appointment with the obstetrician. After giving a brief medical history, I was taken to an examining room where I was asked to leave a urine sample. I was weighed in at 112 pounds, a gain of two. My blood pressure was taken, and the nurse attempted to hear the fetal heartbeat. She was unsuccessful. I was disturbed by this and immediately thought there was something wrong. She quickly assured me it was difficult to hear the heartbeat this early.

WEEK 11

WEEK 12

This week I purchased my first pair of maternity pants with adjustable snaps on the waistband to accommodate my growing waistline (wonderful when you go out to eat). I've subscribed to various child care magazines. I think I'd like to nurse my baby.

YOUR BABY

Your baby is now approximately 3 inches long and weighs about an ounce. Though still incredibly small, he is completely formed. Features are becoming more distinct as fingers, toes, ears, and eyelids form. It is now possible to tell if you're carrying a boy or a girl.

YOUR BODY

It's so unlike you to cry over a sad movie. And taking a nap—you, the human dynamo who could live on four hours sleep a night? And then there is that pulling, nagging pain in your lower abdomen that just won't quit. What's going on anyway?

Early pregnancy is full of changes. Hormonal changes are responsible for your emotional highs and lows and for your fatigue. Both will soon pass. As your uterus grows and as its walls stretch, you often feel a slight cramping or pulling pain. As long as both are pesty and not sharp, there is nothing to worry about. Next time you visit your doctor, describe these sensations. The doctor will confirm that they are quite normal.

At the beginning of the third month your uterus is about the size of an orange. It will grow to the size of a grapefruit before month's end. You may be able to feel or even see a slight bulge above your pubic bone. Your waistline has gotten thicker in response to this growth, and some of your clothes aren't comfortable anymore.

The placenta is completely mature and functioning at top capacity, acting as your baby's lungs, kidneys, liver, digestive tract, and immune system. Your blood volume has increased 30 to 40 percent to nourish you and help make all those routine deliveries to the placenta. This increased blood volume gives you one of pregnancy's best side effects—a glowing face. Now you know why everyone has been commenting on how healthy you look. Tender gums, increased saliva, increased vaginal discharge, minor indigestion, and heartburn are all signs that changes are taking place. You are probably still quite thirsty, and you may be perspiring more than usual, too. Many of these changes relate to your body's increased fluid requirement.

FABULOUS FLUIDS

Water—containing no calories and providing few, if any, nutrients—is second only to air in its importance to life. Water is part of every living cell and essential for every process in the body. Developing babies live in and "breathe" water long before they take their first breath of air.

As your pregnancy weight increases, so does the amount of water in your body. Some women gain as much as 11 pounds of fluid, along with four cups amniotic fluid and about a quart and a half of extra circulating blood. To meet this need for additional fluids, you should drink at least ten 8-ounce glasses of liquid a day.

You can assume that two to four cups of fluid will be found in the foods you eat, many of which, like fruits, contain a lot of water. The rest comes from beverages—tap water, bottled water, milk, fruit juice, fruit punch, and carbonated fruit drinks are all good sources. But don't count coffee, tea, soft drinks, or alcohol. Coffee and tea are diuretics, which make you lose fluid. Alcohol causes dehydration not hydration, and it is potentially harmful to your developing baby. Soft drinks are high in sugar and displace more nutritious choices.

Stick with the basics. Each day drink:

3 to 4 glasses of low-fat milk
1 to 2 glasses of fruit juice
2 to 4 glasses of water

Thirst serves as the body's barometer of water need. Most women find themselves very thirsty during the first trimester and while they are nursing. Thirst is a natural signal that your body needs additional fluid. It's smart to drink one or two more glasses of fluid each day than your thirst tells you to drink. By the time the brain signals you through the thirst mechanism, your body water is already low.

Activity is a major factor that increases your daily fluid need, and pregnant women have a great deal of internal activity going on. Your normal body functions, along with the additional energy needed to support your baby's growth, will generate a good deal of heat. That's why pregnant women are never cold!

Body water acts as a coolant, the same way water cools the engine of your car. When excessive heat needs to be removed from the body, perspiration is released through the skin. Next time you are sitting at your desk and suddenly feel beads of sweat on your forehead or upper lip—quite common at this point in pregnancy— you can smile and imagine the important construction work that is going on in your uterus right now.

THE BEST BEVERAGES

All of the following are good sources of fluid and key nutrients. **Drink these beverages frequently:**

Low-fat or skim milk (3 to 4 cups a day)	An excellent source of calcium. Contains all the nutrients but less fat than regular milk.
Fruit juice (1 to 2 cups a day)	An excellent source of vitamin C.
Water (2 to 4 cups a day)	An excellent source of fluid. Usually contains small amounts of essential minerals, too.
Bottled water or mineral water (as desired)	Lightly mineralized water that may be flavored and/or carbonated is a good water substitute. Can be mixed with fruit juice.

All of the following are good sources of fluids, but they provide very few key nutrients. **Drink these beverages occasionally:**

Fruit punch and sparklers	Often sweetened and diluted with water; less nutritious than 100% fruit juice.

Soda	Contain calories from sugar and little else. Will displace more nourishing choices.
Diet soda	Contains artificial sweeteners that are safe in moderate amounts but offer no nutrients and displace other more nourishing choices.
Tea and coffee	Contains caffeine and should be limited during pregnancy. Acts as a diuretic, causing water loss.

All these may be harmful to your developing baby. **Avoid them.**

| Beer, wine, and other alcoholic drinks. | Alcohol will dehydrate rather than hydrate the body. |

YOUR DIET: VITAMIN C

Vitamin C is especially important during your baby's development because it has so many functions in the body. It helps in the development of collagen, a protein that gives structure to bones, cartilage, muscles, and blood vessels. Vitamin C also helps the body to utilize iron and calcium, produce blood cells, and develop the proper immune response, and it aids in wound healing.

Food consumption studies show that most pregnant women get enough vitamin C each day. The Food and Nutrition Board of the National Academy of Sciences recommends 70 milligrams a day— 10 milligrams more than when you are not pregnant. It is simple to get this much vitamin C through food.

You already know that it is important to eat five servings of fruits and vegetables each day. Simply select two that are good sources of vitamin C. You've also learned this month that fluids are important to your overall health. Orange juice is a beverage most people enjoy, and it is an excellent source of vitamin C.

Other juices, like apple and grape juice, which are not natural sources of vitamin C, are frequently fortified so that a serving becomes an excellent source. Drink juice as a beverage with your meals. This not only provides vitamin C but additionally aids in the absorption of iron from other foods eaten at that same meal. (You'll learn more about iron in Month 4.) Though most breads and cereals have little or no vitamin C, fortified ready-to-eat cereal usually contains 25 percent or more of your daily need. Check the label on your favorite cereal to see if it is fortified.

Because vitamin C can be easily destroyed in your kitchen, it is important to store and cook foods with vitamin C correctly:

• Eat fruits and vegetables raw whenever possible.
• Steam or microwave vegetables to preserve the vitamin C.
• Cook potatoes in their skin.
• Refrigerate vitamin C–rich juices in a covered opaque pitcher. Don't leave the juice sitting on the kitchen table in the sunlight.
• Do not soak cut-up fruits and vegetables in water before cooking or eating.

In some circumstances it might be necessary for you to take a vitamin C supplement: if you are pregnant with twins; if you are a heavy smoker or were shortly before you became pregnant; if you do not eat fruits and vegetables. If you have never eaten many fruits and vegetables, now is the time to change your eating habits so that you can take the best possible care of yourself and your baby during pregnancy. Your doctor will help you decide if you need a vitamin C supplement. In those special cases where it is needed, the National Academy of Sciences recommends a 50-milligram supplement daily. During pregnancy it is important not to take large amounts of vitamin C as a supplement. Too much of one nutrient can interfere with the functions of other nutrients and may even disturb the delivery of nutrients via the placenta to your developing baby. (See "Give Some Thought to Megadoses," in Month 2.)

EXCELLENT SOURCES OF VITAMIN C

Baked potato
Broccoli
Brussels sprouts
Cantaloupe
Cauliflower
Collard greens
Grapefruit
Grapefruit juice
Guava
Orange
Orange juice

Papaya
Persimmon
Pineapple (fresh)
Red and green peppers
Spinach
Strawberries
Tangerine
Tomato
Tomato juice
Watermelon

GIVE SOME THOUGHT TO CRAVINGS

Pregnancy, pickles, and ice cream seem to go hand in hand. Every woman has a story of a food she craved during pregnancy or another that she just hated and couldn't bear to go near. Both situations are common. Studies have shown that over 80 percent of all pregnant women crave certain foods, while 50 percent find other foods intolerable. Fruits and juice, ice cream, sherbet, milk, candy, sweets, and fish are some of the foods women crave, whereas some may avoid coffee, fried foods, meats, greens, and sauces with oregano. Changes in taste and smell that occur during pregnancy along with beliefs passed on from generation to generation may explain some of these choices. Pregnancy cravings baffle most experts. They agree that cravings happen, but they aren't quite sure why.

Some pregnant women even crave nonfood substances—dirt, clay, laundry starch, ice, burned matches. This is called "pica" and could be potentially harmful to both the pregnant woman and her baby. Many of these nonfood items contain harmful substances that were never intended to be eaten.

The best advice: *Indulge your cravings, but don't go overboard. Stay away from those foods that bother you. Talk to your doctor if you are eating nonfood substances.*

DAILY FOOD GUIDE TO
KEY NUTRIENTS NEEDED
DURING PREGNANCY

To be sure that you get all the key nutrients you and your developing baby need each day, follow this daily food guide. Each day have:

2 to 3 servings (4 to 6 ounces)	protein-rich foods
4 servings	calcium-rich food
5 servings	fruits and vegetables
5 or more servings	breads, cereals, grains (whole grain and enriched varie- ties)

TRACKING KEY NUTRIENTS ON THE
PREGNANCY FOOD CHECKLIST

1. Record a sample day during each week of pregnancy.
2. Calculate the amount of each key nutrient eaten that day.
3. If you fall short of any of the key nutrients, change your food choices to be sure you've included all the key nutrients you and your developing baby need.

PREGNANCY FOOD CHECKLIST
Month 3, Week 1

	CAL	PRO (G)	VIT C (MG)	FOL (MCG)	CA (MG)	IR (MG)
BREAKFAST:						
Subtotal	—	—	—	—	—	—
SNACK:						
Subtotal	—	—	—	—	—	—
LUNCH:						
Subtotal	—	—	—	—	—	—
SNACK:						
Subtotal	—	—	—	—	—	—
DINNER:						
Subtotal	—	—	—	—	—	—
SNACK:						
Subtotal	—	—	—	—	—	—
Daily Totals	—	—	—	—	—	—
Daily Nutrient Goals	2200	60	70	400	1200	30

PREGNANCY FOOD CHECKLIST
Month 3, Week 2

	CAL	PRO (G)	VIT C (MG)	FOL (MCG)	CA (MG)	IR (MG)
BREAKFAST:						
Subtotal	—	—	—	—	—	—
SNACK:						
Subtotal	—	—	—	—	—	—
LUNCH:						
Subtotal	—	—	—	—	—	—
SNACK:						
Subtotal	—	—	—	—	—	—
DINNER:						
Subtotal	—	—	—	—	—	—
SNACK:						
Subtotal	—	—	—	—	—	—
Daily Totals	—	—	—	—	—	—
Daily Nutrient Goals	2200	60	70	400	1200	30

PREGNANCY FOOD CHECKLIST
Month 3, Week 3

	CAL	PRO (G)	VIT C (MG)	FOL (MCG)	CA (MG)	IR (MG)
BREAKFAST:						
Subtotal	—	—	—	—	—	—
SNACK:						
Subtotal	—	—	—	—	—	—
LUNCH:						
Subtotal	—	—	—	—	—	—
SNACK:						
Subtotal	—	—	—	—	—	—
DINNER:						
Subtotal	—	—	—	—	—	—
SNACK:						
Subtotal	—	—	—	—	—	—
Daily Totals	—	—	—	—	—	—
Daily Nutrient Goals	2200	60	70	400	1200	30

PREGNANCY FOOD CHECKLIST
Month 3, Week 4

	CAL	PRO (G)	VIT C (MG)	FOL (MCG)	CA (MG)	IR (MG)
BREAKFAST:						
Subtotal	—	—	—	—	—	—
SNACK:						
Subtotal	—	—	—	—	—	—
LUNCH:						
Subtotal	—	—	—	—	—	—
SNACK:						
Subtotal	—	—	—	—	—	—
DINNER:						
Subtotal	—	—	—	—	—	—
SNACK:						
Subtotal	—	—	—	—	—	—
Daily Totals	—	—	—	—	—	—
Daily Nutrient Goals	2200	60	70	400	1200	30

<u>MONTH 3</u>

Month _____ Year _____

Your feelings:

_____

_____

_____

_____

_____

_____

Your questions for your doctor or nurse-midwife:

_____

_____

_____

_____

_____

_____

_____

_____

_____

_____

_____

THE

SECOND

TRIMESTER

MONTH 4

A Mother's Journal

WEEK 13

WEEK 14

This week I had my second prenatal appointment. I have gained two pounds, and the nurse heard the fetal heartbeat. I told the doctor I have not had any morning sickness yet. He said vomiting usually occurs only in the first trimester. If I've gotten to this point without an episode of vomiting, I probably won't be bothered with it in the future.

WEEK 15

I have more energy and am urinating less frequently. I must be entering the easy part of pregnancy.

WEEK 16

YOUR BABY

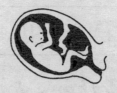

During this month your baby grows to about eight to ten inches long, about half the length she will be at birth. She now weighs about 6 ounces and you can feel her kicking, stretching, and moving around. Your baby can now make a fist, frown, open its mouth, and squint its eyes. All major organs and body structures are formed, and the foundation of baby's skeleton is in place. From here on, your baby will simply grow bigger and stronger as time goes on.

YOUR BODY

You've just begun the second trimester of your pregnancy, months 4 to 6. This is the easy part. You look good, you feel good, and you're happy. Most of the discomforts of the first three months have passed, and your old energy level is back. This isn't going to be so hard after all!

The most exciting thing to happen this month is that you will begin to feel your baby move! In first pregnancies this usually occurs around the end of the fourth month, but there is a great deal of variation, so don't be concerned if your baby doesn't make himself noticed right on schedule.

The first sensation of movement is so faint you may miss it unless you know what you are looking for. Some women describe it as a fluttering or shimmering sensation in the lower abdomen. Others say it is as if someone were blowing a fine stream of bubbles inside them.

Your prepregnancy shape is noticeably disappearing, and it won't be long before you'll be in maternity clothes full time. You may have a headache or a nosebleed. This is just a sign that your body is adjusting to its increased blood volume and vessel tension. Neither is a serious problem, but do tell your doctor if either occurs. By the end of the month your total weight gain will probably be about six to eight pounds, but this also varies a great deal.

WEIGHTY MATTERS

Because our society puts such a premium on being thin, many women have difficulty feeling comfortable about gaining weight during pregnancy. Intellectually, you know that this weight gain is important, but emotionally, as you see the numbers go up on the scale and watch your enlarging shape, you get nervous.

Pregnancy weight gain is one of the most positive predictors of pregnancy outcome. Women who eat well throughout pregnancy and gain the appropriate amount of weight are more likely to have healthy babies.

During the first trimester your weight gain will average 2 to 4 pounds. During the rest of pregnancy, you'll gain an average of ¾ to 1 pound a week. Weight gain during the second and third trimesters varies from woman to woman and from pregnancy to pregnancy but generally shows a gradual and steady increase with no sudden gains or losses. You'll hardly notice your weight gain in the first three months, but during the second trimester the weight gain will become obvious as your blood volume, your breast tissue, and your baby's size increase. In the third trimester most of the weight gain will occur in your baby, which triples in weight during the last growth spurt before birth.

Most experts recommend that expectant mothers gain between 24 and 28 pounds. The illustration on page 56 gives you an idea of how that weight adds up. Recent statistics compiled by the National Center for Health Statistics showed that women who gained between 26 and 35 pounds had the healthiest babies. This and other convincing evidence on the benefits of adequate weight gain during pregnancy have resulted in new weight-gain recommendations based on prepregnancy weight. Women of normal weight before pregnancy are encouraged to gain between 24 and 35 pounds during pregnancy. For those who were underweight before pregnancy gaining up to 40 pounds is beneficial. For women who were overweight before pregnancy, weight gains between 24 and 29 pounds are adequate.

On pages 57, 58, and 59 are three average weight-gain charts for women who are normal, underweight, and overweight at the start of pregnancy. You can use the chart that is appropriate for you and plot your own weight gain. The table "Estimating Prepregnancy Weight

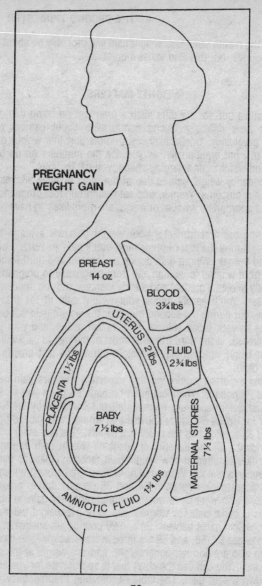

PREGNANCY
WEIGHT GAIN

BREAST
14 oz

BLOOD
3¾ lbs

UTERUS 2 lbs

PLACENTA 1½ lbs

FLUID
2¾ lbs

BABY
7½ lbs

MATERNAL STORES
7½ lbs

AMNIOTIC FLUID 1¾ lbs

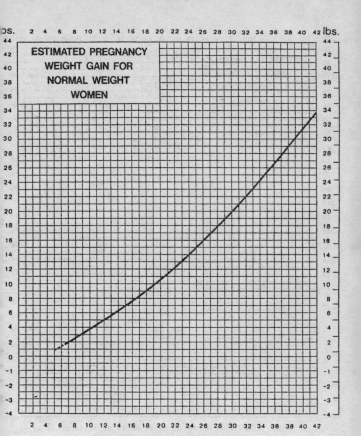

ESTIMATED PREGNANCY
WEIGHT GAIN FOR
NORMAL WEIGHT
WOMEN

WEEKS OF PREGNANCY

adapted from Brown, J.E. University of Minnesota, 1986

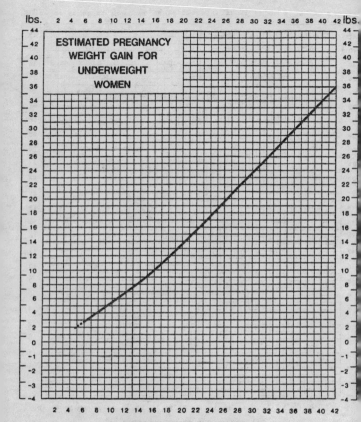

lbs.

ESTIMATED PREGNANCY WEIGHT GAIN FOR UNDERWEIGHT WOMEN

WEEKS OF PREGNANCY

adapted from Brown, J.E. University of Minnesota 1986

58

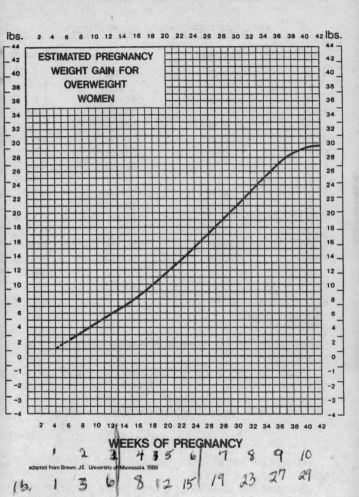

ESTIMATED PREGNANCY WEIGHT GAIN FOR OVERWEIGHT WOMEN

WEEKS OF PREGNANCY

adapted from Brown, J.E. University of Minnesota, 1986

	1	2	3	4	5	6	7	8	9	10
lb.	1	3	6	8	12	15	19	23	27	29

59

ESTIMATING PREPREGNANCY WEIGHT STATUS*

Height**	Underweight	Normal	Overweight
4' 8"	< 89	89–109	110–129
4' 9"	< 91	91–111	112–131
4'10"	< 94	94–114	115–135
4'11"	< 96	96–117	118–139
5'	< 99	99–121	122–143
5' 1"	<102	102–124	125–147
5' 2"	<105	105–128	129–152
5' 3"	<109	109–133	134–157
5' 4"	<112	112–137	138–162
5' 5"	<116	116–142	143–167
5' 6"	<120	120–146	147–173
5' 7"	<123	123–151	152–178
5' 8"	<127	127–155	156–183
5' 9"	<130	130–159	160–188
5'10"	<134	134–163	164–193
5'11"	<137	137–167	168–197
6'	<140	140–171	172–202
6' 1"	<143	143–175	176–207

*Weight without clothes
**Without shoes

Status,'' above, will help you determine which weight-gain chart is for you.

Keep in mind that charts like these are intended to be used as a guide, not followed like a rule. For each woman and each pregnancy, weight gain will be slightly different. Your weight should generally follow the trend on the chart, but don't worry if it varies slightly.

A WORD ABOUT TESTS

Two tests that may be done in the fourth month of pregnancy are ultrasound and amniocentesis.

Ultrasound uses sound waves to take a picture (sonogram) of the baby in the uterus. This sonogram shows the size and shape of the baby. Sometimes a Polaroid shot is taken of the sonogram as baby's first picture.

For most pregnant women the sonogram provides reassurance that the baby's growth and development are normal. If a problem is diagnosed with ultrasound, steps can be taken to treat it. While this test is not essential for most low-risk pregnancies, the doctor may suggest it to help estimate the due date or to confirm a multiple pregnancy. Later on in pregnancy, ultrasound testing may be used to determine the size and position of the baby.

Amniocentesis is a procedure in which a small amount of amniotic fluid is removed from the uterus and checked in a lab. A large number of birth defects can be diagnosed this way. Usually done in the fourth month of pregnancy, this test is used routinely for most women over the age of thirty-five and in others where there is believed to be a risk of birth defect.

Maternal serum alpha-fetoprotein screening (MS-AFP) tests the blood level of a protein made by the baby's liver and passed into the mother's blood. A certain amount of this protein is a sign that the baby is developing normally. Very high or very low levels of this protein may be a sign of possible birth defects so that further testing is done. Some states require this test be done.

YOUR DIET: IRON

During a normal pregnancy you will need over 1,000 milligrams of iron to meet the growth needs of your baby; to allow the baby to store iron in his tissues for use in the first few months after birth; to support the growth of the placenta; and to allow your blood supply to increase. The demand for iron is so great that it is estimated that as many as one half of all pregnant women have less than desirable amounts of iron in their body. It will take two years of eating well after pregnancy to restore your iron reserves. If your pregnancies are spaced closer than this, if you have more than one baby at a time, or if your iron stores are lower than normal, you would be at greater risk for anemia.

At the beginning of your pregnancy, there was approximately 2.2 grams of iron in your body—about the weight of a dime. Though this amount may seem tiny, iron is one of the most essential elements. It makes up part of the red blood cell hemoglobin (*heme* = iron; *globin* = protein) which is essential for the transport and use of oxygen in the body.

Your need for iron doubles during pregnancy. The Food and Nutrition Board of the National Academy of Sciences recommends 30 milligrams a day. Getting this amount through food is a real challenge. Most women are unable to get adequate amounts of iron from food. Food surveys estimate that normal intakes range from 10 to 17 milligrams a day. For that reason, most physicians encourage their patients to take an iron supplement in the second and third trimester. The National Academy recommends a 30-milligram iron supplement starting around the twelfth week of pregnancy, along with the consumption of iron-rich foods.

A good goal would be to try to consume 15 milligrams of iron a day through iron-rich food sources and take the iron supplement recommended by your doctor.

You are probably thinking, if my iron supplement gives me 30 milligrams a day and the recommendation is 30 milligrams, why should I worry about iron-rich food at all? Food sources of iron are important because the iron found in food is more efficiently absorbed than the iron available in a supplement.

The absorption of iron is a complicated process. It depends on your sex, your need for iron, whether the iron is in a food or a supplement, and when the iron is taken. Women absorb twice as much iron as men because they have lower iron stores to start with and because their need is greater due to monthly menstrual loss. Pregnant women absorb more iron than nonpregnant women because their need is even greater and it steadily increases as pregnancy goes on.

Iron in food is absorbed better than iron from a supplement. The ability to absorb and use iron from different foods varies. The iron in meat, poultry, and fish is absorbed and used more easily than iron in other foods. If you include one of these animal products in a meal, the availability of iron from all the other foods you eat at that meal is increased. Including vitamin C in a meal also increases iron absorption. Drinking orange juice instead of water at dinner will double the amount of iron absorbed; drinking coffee or tea will cut your iron absorption in half. The body absorbs iron most efficiently when stores are low or during growth. Pregnancy is a period of rapid growth, so you absorb iron optimally. Pasta, white rice, and most breads are enriched with iron. Whole grains naturally contain the mineral. Though these are not the best sources, they do contribute a significant amount of iron to your overall intake. The same holds true for fortified ready-to-eat or instant cereals.

Even though your body will not absorb all the iron in your iron supplement, it is nonetheless important for you to take your supplement as directed. When you read the label, it may seem like the supplement your doctor recommended has an enormous amount of iron in it. For example, if you are taking one 150-milligram tablet of ferrous sulfate daily, are you really taking 150 milligrams of iron? No. The supplement is a compound called ferrous sulfate; iron makes up only 20 percent of the combination—in other words, the tablet provides 30 milligrams of iron, the recommended supplement level. A 150-milligram tablet of ferrous gluconate provides 12 percent, or 18 milligrams, of iron. Ferrous fumarate gives 35 percent iron, or 48 milligrams. To most efficiently absorb the iron from your supplement, take it without food in the evening before bed.

IS IT SAFE TO EAT LIVER?

Everyone knows that liver is an outstanding source of iron. But today many people are worried about eating this low-fat, high-protein organ meat. They are concerned about its high cholesterol content and its role in detoxifying waste products in an animal's body.

The liver is the place in the body where cholesterol is made, so it makes sense that it would be high in cholesterol. It also does play a major role in ridding the body of harmful wastes. But interestingly it does not store these toxins but helps the body excrete them or store them in fat. The fat around a steak is more likely to contain toxins and pollutants than a slice of calves' liver.

A sensible recommendation: *If you like liver, enjoy it once or twice a month.*

GOOD SOURCES OF IRON

Baked beans	Meat
Blueberries	Peanuts
Chick-peas	Peas
Eggs	Poultry
Enriched breads and cereals	Prune juice
Fish	Prunes
Kidney beans	Raisins
Lima beans	Spinach

GIVE SOME THOUGHT TO CAFFEINE

Caffeine is a chemical stimulant found in coffee, tea, soda, cocoa, chocolate, and prescription and nonprescription drugs. People have used it for centuries to get a lift, and today people of every culture regularly consume a caffeine-containing food or drink.

Approximately 99 percent of the caffeine ingested is absorbed, and it freely crosses the placenta. The usual half-life of caffeine—the time required for the body to eliminate one-half the amount taken in—is three to seven hours in adult nonsmokers. For pregnant women this time increases to eighteen to twenty hours.

Some animal studies showed that caffeine could be harmful to developing offspring, but in those cases the test subjects were force-fed caffeine equaling fifty-six to eighty-seven cups of coffee a day. When caffeine was given in more normal amounts no problems occurred.

This and other evidence has led experts to agree that there is no proof that *moderate* amounts of caffeine during pregnancy will harm your baby. Soda, coffee, and tea contribute the most caffeine while chocolate and cocoa contain very little.

There are ways to cut down on caffeine without cutting out beverages you enjoy. Tea has less caffeine, cup for cup, than coffee. Weak tea has less than a strong brew. Soda containing caffeine must list it on the label; select caffeine-free choices. Drip coffee has the most caffeine, instant the least. Making coffee from half decaf and half regular reduces the caffeine in a cup to that of a cup of weakly brewed tea. Mixtures of coffee and grain (caffeine-reduced) are another interesting alternative to try.

Remember that caffeine-containing drinks and foods make no significant nutritional contribution to your diet. They are simply flavorful, often pleasurable choices. If you decide to cut back or cut them out, you are in no way compromising on key nutrients.

The best advice: *Limit caffeine-containing drinks to two a day and spread out your intake throughout the day to prevent high concentrations in your body and to give your body time to clear the caffeine before you have more.*

DAILY FOOD GUIDE TO
KEY NUTRIENTS NEEDED
DURING PREGNANCY

To be sure that you get all the key nutrients you and your developing baby need each day, follow this daily food guide. Each day have:

2 to 3 servings (4 to 6 ounces)	protein-rich foods
4 servings	calcium-rich food
5 servings	fruits and vegetables
5 or more servings	breads, cereals, grains (whole grain and enriched varieties)

TRACKING KEY NUTRIENTS ON THE
PREGNANCY FOOD CHECKLIST

1. Record a sample day during each week of pregnancy.
2. Calculate the amount of each key nutrient eaten that day.
3. If you fall short of any of the key nutrients, change your food choices to be sure you've included all the key nutrients you and your developing baby need.

PREGNANCY FOOD CHECKLIST
Month 4, Week 1

	CAL	PRO (G)	VIT C (MG)	FOL (MCG)	CA (MG)	IR (MG)
BREAKFAST:						
Subtotal	——	——	——	——	——	——
SNACK:						
Subtotal	——	——	——	——	——	——
LUNCH:						
Subtotal	——	——	——	——	——	——
SNACK:						
Subtotal	——	——	——	——	——	——
DINNER:						
Subtotal	——	——	——	——	——	——
SNACK:						
Subtotal	——	——	——	——	——	——
Daily Totals	——	——	——	——	——	——
Daily Nutrient Goals	2200	60	70	400	1200	30

PREGNANCY FOOD CHECKLIST
Month 4, Week 2

	CAL	PRO (G)	VIT C (MG)	FOL (MCG)	CA (MG)	IR (MG)
BREAKFAST:						
Subtotal	——	——	——	——	——	——
SNACK:						
Subtotal	——	——	——	——	——	——
LUNCH:						
Subtotal	——	——	——	——	——	——
SNACK:						
Subtotal	——	——	——	——	——	——
DINNER:						
Subtotal	——	——	——	——	——	——
SNACK:						
Subtotal	——	——	——	——	——	——
Daily Totals	——	——	——	——	——	——
Daily Nutrient Goals	2200	60	70	400	1200	30

PREGNANCY FOOD CHECKLIST
Month 4, Week 3

	CAL	PRO (G)	VIT C (MG)	FOL (MCG)	CA (MG)	IR (MG)
BREAKFAST:						
Subtotal	——	——	——	——	——	——
SNACK:						
Subtotal	——	——	——	——	——	——
LUNCH:						
Subtotal	——	——	——	——	——	——
SNACK:						
Subtotal	——	——	——	——	——	——
DINNER:						
Subtotal	——	——	——	——	——	——
SNACK:						
Subtotal	——	——	——	——	——	——
Daily Totals	——	——	——	——	——	——
Daily Nutrient Goals	2200	60	70	400	1200	30

PREGNANCY FOOD CHECKLIST
Month 4, Week 4

	CAL	PRO (G)	VIT C (MG)	FOL (MCG)	CA (MG)	IR (MG)
BREAKFAST:						
Subtotal	——	——	——	——	——	——
SNACK:						
Subtotal	——	——	——	——	——	——
LUNCH:						
Subtotal	——	——	——	——	——	——
SNACK:						
Subtotal	——	——	——	——	——	——
DINNER:						
Subtotal	——	——	——	——	——	——
SNACK:						
Subtotal	——	——	——	——	——	——
Daily Totals	——	——	——	——	——	——
Daily Nutrient Goals	2200	60	70	400	1200	30

MONTH 4

Month _____ Year _____

Your feelings:

_____

_____

_____

_____

_____

_____

Your questions for your doctor or nurse-midwife:

_____

_____

_____

_____

_____

_____

_____

_____

_____

_____

_____

MONTH 5

A Mother's Journal

WEEK 17

I had my third appointment with the doctor. Since my last visit I've gained 3 pounds. The nurse heard the baby's heartbeat. Initially my blood pressure was a bit high. The nurse told me to rest on my left side and she'd recheck my pressure in ten minutes. The result of the second check was closer to normal.

WEEK 18

WEEK 19

WEEK 20

YOUR BABY

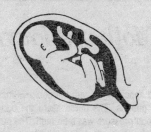

Your baby has established his own pattern of sleeping, turning, sucking, and kicking and has found a favorite position in your uterus. Your child's eyebrows and eyelashes grow, as does soft downy hair, called lanugo, which covers his body but will be shed before birth. Lungs are practicing how to breathe as they inhale and exhale amniotic fluid. Your baby weighs about a pound and is a foot long.

YOUR BODY

Your pregnancy is almost half over. You've gained enough weight—somewhere between 11 and 16 pounds—to shift your center of gravity. You compensate by leaning back when you walk or stand, and this causes backache. Sit with your lower back supported, sleep on your side on a firm mattress, and wear low-heeled shoes.

You may feel breathless. This comes from a change in your circulation pattern and from increased pressure on your diaphragm as your baby grows larger.

You may also notice changes in your skin. Your nipples and areola (the skin around the nipples) may darken, and a dark vertical line (linea nigra) from belly button to pubic hair may appear; both fade soon after delivery. Stretch marks (striae) may appear on your belly, thighs, and breasts. They will fade and be much less noticeable after delivery, too. All of your blood vessels have become dilated due to the influence of extra hormones, making them far more noticeable under the skin. This is not unusual, and the effect is only temporary.

Congestion in the veins of the ear canal produces the same feeling that you get in your ears when flying in the pressurized cabin of a plane or after swimming. In some women the congestion persists until delivery; in others it comes and goes.

BEING CAREFUL

During pregnancy you are more susceptible to food-borne illness (food poisoning), so it is important to handle food carefully. Some seven million Americans suffer from food-borne illness every year. Why? Because, at the right temperature, organisms you can't see, smell, or taste can multiply to millions in a few short hours. In large numbers they cause illness. Experts estimate that if people applied a few simple rules for handling food safely, they could eliminate 85 percent of all cases of food-borne illness.

Here are some suggestions for handling food at the supermarket:

Select:
- Clean, unbruised fruits and vegetables
- Cheese, butter, margarine, milk, and yogurt in clean, unopened containers or wrappers
- Clean, uncracked eggs
- Cans without dents, rust, or dirty labels
- Cold, solidly frozen foods in clean, undamaged packages
- Fresh meat, fish, and poultry without off odors in packages that are not dripping
- Cereal, bread, pasta, rice, and beans in unbroken bags or boxes

Never:
- Sample food from an opened package left lying on the shelf
- Leave groceries sitting in a hot car while you do other errands

In your kitchen it is easy to keep foods safe:

- Keep it clean.
- Keep it hot, or keep it cold.
- Keep cooked foods and raw foods separate during preparation.

Remember: clean hands plus clean utensils equal clean food—a simple fact that is often ignored. Wash your hands, countertops, cutting boards, stirring spoons and knives often. Use acrylic cutting boards that are dishwasher safe. If you don't have a dishwasher, you can use soap, water, and friction (scrubbing) to do the same job. Don't use the same cutting board and knife to trim meat for dinner and then to make a tossed salad. That's a perfect way to transmit bacteria from one food to another.

To maintain freshness, quality, and safety in your kitchen:

- Buy the amount of food you can use in a reasonable time. Large quantities are no bargain if they spoil or grow stale.
- Defrost frozen food in the refrigerator or in the microwave; use it within twenty-four hours. Defrosting dinner on the kitchen counter invites the growth of harmful bacteria.
- Refrigerate leftovers promptly and use them in two to three days. If mold appears, do not cut it away and use the rest of the food; throw away the food. Mold is like a flower: you see the blossoms, but the roots are anchored deep in the food.
- Store raw foods below cooked foods in the refrigerator to prevent dripping from the raw to the cooked.
- *Never taste food that you think may have spoiled. When in doubt, throw it out.*

GIVE SOME THOUGHT TO SKIPPING CERTAIN FOODS WHILE YOU ARE PREGNANT

All of the following foods may carry harmful levels of bacteria or other organisms, contain heavy metals like lead or mercury, or be contaminated with pollutants. If you consume these foods in sufficient amounts, they could cause food-borne illness in you and possibly affect the development of your unborn baby:

- Cheese made from unpasteurized milk
- Fresh stream water
- Game
- Raw milk
- Raw or cooked-rare meat, fish, or poultry
- Raw or soft-cooked eggs
- Raw shellfish

The best advice: *Don't eat these foods while you are pregnant.*

A WORD ABOUT TESTS

It is recommended that all women be tested for glucose tolerance during pregnancy. Glucose tolerance is your body's ability to handle sugars and starches. Your doctor will give you a glucose tolerance test early in your pregnancy. If the results are normal, the test will be repeated during the twenty-fourth to twenty-eighth week of pregnancy.

If the glucose challenge test results are questionable, as they are in about one-third of all women, you will be given a more sensitive glucose tolerance test. This will determine whether or not you have gestational diabetes.

Two to three percent of all pregnant women develop gestational diabetes. This happens when women become temporarily resistant to insulin during pregnancy. Your body needs insulin to use sugar and starch normally. Early diagnosis of gestational diabetes and proper care can prevent medical problems for you and your baby.

Most women with gestational diabetes can control it with diet changes. Your doctor will tell you how to do this and may also refer you to a registered dietitian (RD) or a certified diabetes educator (CDE) for more help. In almost all cases the gestational diabetes disappears after delivery.

YOUR DIET: CALCIUM

You know that calcium is important for strong bones and teeth, but you might be surprised to find out that this essential mineral also helps control the heartbeat and transmit nerve messages, and it aids in blood clotting and helps muscles contract. A 120-pound woman has about 2½ pounds of calcium stored in her body. Most of this calcium is in her bones and teeth, but some circulates in the blood or is held in the body's soft tissue.

During pregnancy your need for calcium increases. Not only are you protecting yourself from osteoporosis (adult bone thinning) but you are also providing all the calcium your unborn baby needs to form strong bones and teeth. Though it is highly unlikely that your baby will be born with teeth showing, all of the tooth buds, for both the baby teeth and the permanent teeth, will be in place at birth.

The need for calcium is greatest in the last trimester of pregnancy when the baby's growth is most rapid. Your baby draws 200 to 300 milligrams of calcium a day from your body's supply, accumulating

25,000 milligrams before birth; all of this calcium is supplied by you. You need to replace your body stores as well as continually supply calcium to your baby. The easiest way to do this is by eating calcium-rich foods. The Food and Nutrition Board of the National Academy of Sciences recommends 1,200 milligrams of calcium daily, throughout pregnancy and breast-feeding.

To translate this recommendation into foods you can use the "300 rule." Assume you will get a total of 300 milligrams of calcium daily, in small amounts, when you eat a variety of foods. Additionally assume that one cup of milk, one cup of yogurt, and 1½ ounces of hard cheese will each provide approximately 300 milligrams of calcium. Thus, by eating three calcium-rich dairy foods each day, in addition to eating a wide variety of other good foods, you will meet the experts' recommendation of 1,200 milligrams a day.

If you experience a tummy ache, bloating, gas, or diarrhea shortly after you've had milk or foods containing milk, you may be *lactose intolerant*—unable to digest the milk sugar, *lactose,* because you do not have enough of the digestive enzyme *lactase*.

If you have this problem, there are still many ways to meet your calcium requirement during pregnancy. Try smaller servings of milk—a half or quarter cup rather than a full glass. Chocolate milk, cooked milk in the form of pudding or custard, and ice cream may cause no discomfort. Fermented dairy foods like yogurt, kefir, and buttermilk may have less lactose. Hard cheeses have little or none. There are also calcium-rich nondairy foods you can eat regularly. (See Sources of Calcium, page 78).

If you can't drink milk, try yogurt, kefir, buttermilk, hard cheese, cottage cheese, pudding, custard, creamed soup, ice cream, or chocolate milk.

Most experts feel that a pregnant woman should get at least half her daily calcium from food. Calcium-rich foods provide other important nutrients, like protein, riboflavin (a B vitamin), phosphorus (a mineral), and vitamin D, along with calcium. That means you should be eating two to three calcium-rich foods each day and taking a supplement of 600 milligrams of calcium. Your doctor will help you decide if you need a calcium supplement. If you do, take it in the evening with a small glass of milk to achieve maximum absorption. *Do not take your calcium supplement and iron supplement at the same time.*

THE STUFF MYTHS ARE MADE OF

"For every baby you lose a tooth"

The vision one imagines is that of a baby hammering feverishly at the mother's teeth in order to satisfy his need for calcium. In truth, however, the calcium in your teeth is *inert*—once formed, it cannot be removed from the tooth structure.

The dental problems that occur during pregnancy are usually the result of changes in the saliva and gums, making the teeth more accessible to bacteria. By visiting the dentist regularly and by practicing good dental hygiene you can easily avoid this problem.

TROUBLE SPOTS

Pregnancy-induced Hypertension (PIH)

Formerly known as *toxemia,* PIH occurs in pregnant women who have not previously had high blood pressure. Beside high blood pressure, symptoms of PIH include edema (fluid retention) and protein in the urine (which can be detected in the sample you supply at each routine visit to your doctor). The cause of PIH is unknown, but studies have shown that women who get adequate calcium have a lower incidence of this condition.

More research is needed on the possible relation between calcium and PIH, but in the meantime, getting adequate calcium is important to your baby's development and to your long-range good health. It may also protect you against this trouble spot.

SOURCES OF CALCIUM

EXCELLENT SOURCES

Buttermilk
Calcium-fortified orange juice
Chocolate milk
Hard cheeses
Low-fat milk

Ricotta cheese
Sardines, with bones
Skim milk
Whole milk
Yogurt

GOOD SOURCES

Almonds
American cheese
Broccoli
Collard greens
Cottage cheese
Custard
Fortified ready-to-eat breakfast
  cereal

Ice cream
Pudding
Salmon with bones
Shrimp
Spinach
Tofu (soybean curd)

DAILY FOOD GUIDE TO
KEY NUTRIENTS NEEDED
DURING PREGNANCY

To be sure that you get all the key nutrients you and your developing baby need each day, follow this daily food guide. Each day have:

2 to 3 servings (4 to 6 ounces)	protein-rich foods
4 servings	calcium-rich food
5 servings	fruits and vegetables
5 or more servings	breads, cereals, grains (whole grain and enriched varieties)

TRACKING KEY NUTRIENTS ON THE
PREGNANCY FOOD CHECKLIST

1. Record a sample day during each week of pregnancy.
2. Calculate the amount of each key nutrient eaten that day.
3. If you fall short of any of the key nutrients, change your food choices to be sure you've included all the key nutrients you and your developing baby need.

PREGNANCY FOOD CHECKLIST
Month 5, Week 1

	CAL	PRO (G)	VIT C (MG)	FOL (MCG)	CA (MG)	IR (MG)
BREAKFAST:						
Subtotal	—	—	—	—	—	—
SNACK:						
Subtotal	—	—	—	—	—	—
LUNCH:						
Subtotal	—	—	—	—	—	—
SNACK:						
Subtotal	—	—	—	—	—	—
DINNER:						
Subtotal	—	—	—	—	—	—
SNACK:						
Subtotal	—	—	—	—	—	—
Daily Totals	—	—	—	—	—	—
Daily Nutrient Goals	2200	60	70	400	1200	30

PREGNANCY FOOD CHECKLIST
Month 5, Week 2

	CAL	PRO (G)	VIT C (MG)	FOL (MCG)	CA (MG)	IR (MG)
BREAKFAST:						
Subtotal	—	—	—	—	—	—
SNACK:						
Subtotal	—	—	—	—	—	—
LUNCH:						
Subtotal	—	—	—	—	—	—
SNACK:						
Subtotal	—	—	—	—	—	—
DINNER:						
Subtotal	—	—	—	—	—	—
SNACK:						
Subtotal	—	—	—	—	—	—
Daily Totals	—	—	—	—	—	—
Daily Nutrient Goals	2200	60	70	400	1200	30

PREGNANCY FOOD CHECKLIST
Month 5, Week 3

	CAL	PRO (G)	VIT C (MG)	FOL (MCG)	CA (MG)	IR (MG)
BREAKFAST:						
Subtotal	—	—	—	—	—	—
SNACK:						
Subtotal	—	—	—	—	—	—
LUNCH:						
Subtotal	—	—	—	—	—	—
SNACK:						
Subtotal	—	—	—	—	—	—
DINNER:						
Subtotal	—	—	—	—	—	—
SNACK:						
Subtotal	—	—	—	—	—	—
Daily Totals	—	—	—	—	—	—
Daily Nutrient Goals	2200	60	70	400	1200	30

PREGNANCY FOOD CHECKLIST
Month 5, Week 4

	CAL	PRO (G)	VIT C (MG)	FOL (MCG)	CA (MG)	IR (MG)
BREAKFAST:						
Subtotal	___	___	___	___	___	___
SNACK:						
Subtotal	___	___	___	___	___	___
LUNCH:						
Subtotal	___	___	___	___	___	___
SNACK:						
Subtotal	___	___	___	___	___	___
DINNER:						
Subtotal	___	___	___	___	___	___
SNACK:						
Subtotal	___	___	___	___	___	___
Daily Totals	___	___	___	___	___	___
Daily Nutrient Goals	2200	60	70	400	1200	30

<u>MONTH 5</u>

Month _____ Year _____

Your feelings:

_____
_____
_____
_____
_____
_____

Your questions for your doctor or nurse-midwife:

_____
_____
_____
_____
_____
_____
_____
_____
_____
_____
_____

MONTH 6

A Mother's Journal

WEEK 21

WEEK 22

I could eat constantly. I've gained 14 pounds. I can't truthfully say I gained this weight on fruit and vegetables alone. There have been quite a few brownies, cookies, and bowls of ice cream. I pledge to go easier on the sweets. Whenever I catch a glimpse of myself in a full-length mirror, I'm aghast! I really don't look pregnant; I just look as if I need to go on a diet. I'm tempted to get one of those pregnancy T-shirts with a clever saying on the front.

WEEK 23

I registered for prenatal classes. I'm looking forward to them and curious to see how large the other pregnant women are. It's still hard for me to believe that in three and a half months I'll be a mother. I'm no longer as intimidated as I initially was.

WEEK 24

I feel the baby moving quite a bit, and it is very reassuring.

YOUR BABY

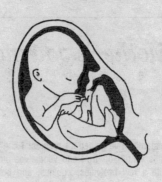

If you could peep inside your uterus you would see a red, wrinkled little person. This withered look will soon change as your baby begins to store more fat under her skin. The inner ear has developed so she can hear and may be startled by loud sounds. Because of this ability to hear, if you talk to your baby throughout pregnancy, she will know and recognize your voice at birth. Your baby now weighs up to two pounds and has grown about two inches since last month.

YOUR BODY

Your baby is kicking or, in quieter moments, actively sucking his thumb. Most mothers can sense when their baby is awake. Every so often a kick may catch you by surprise.

Your silhouette is obviously pregnant. It is not unusual to gain as much as a pound a week from now on. Your baby is growing steadily, and the placenta is becoming thicker and wider to meet the increased demand for nutrients.

Your belly button may pop from internal pressure, but it will recede after delivery. And you may feel as if you've aged: you'll be unable to get up quickly from a sitting position and you may creak when you walk or bend. This is due to the hormone relaxin, which is secreted to relax the ligaments around your pelvis and hips so that they can stretch more easily during labor.

HEARTBURN

As your uterus grows and begins to sandwich your digestive tract between it and your backbone, you may be belching and having heartburn. Heartburn has nothing to do with the heart, though you experience a burning sensation in the middle of your chest.

This happens when a circular muscle between the stomach and esophagus relaxes (opens) and allows acidic stomach contents to splash up onto delicate tissue in the esophagus. Coffee, chocolate, alcohol, foods high in fat, peppermint and spearmint flavors, and smoking tend to relax this muscle. If you end a meal with any of these, like a slice of cheesecake or an after-dinner mint, your chance of having heartburn is greater. Gravity can also aggravate the problem. Eating late at night and lying down after eating can make the problem worse. Skim milk tends to tighten the circular muscle. Try drinking a small glass at the end of each meal and just before bed. Don't use over-the-counter remedies for heartburn before you discuss them with your doctor.

YOUR DIET: SALT—SPRINKLE LIGHTLY

You often hear and read cautions to reduce your salt intake. More precisely, these warnings apply to the mineral sodium, which makes up 40 percent of salt. During certain times in history, salt was scarce and considered very valuable. Today we take this readily available, common seasoning for granted and often use more than ten times the amount we need.

The Food and Nutrition Board of the National Academy of Sciences does not give a daily sodium recommendation specific to pregnancy. Instead the board sets a minimum intake of 500 milligrams. This amount provides an ample supply of sodium for all healthy adults.

Sodium is essential to maintain the fluid balance in the body. During pregnancy your total body fluids increase. It makes sense that the major mineral in that fluid, sodium, must also increase. You'll easily meet this increased need if you eat a varied diet. You get sodium naturally in milk, meat, eggs, and vegetables. In other foods—pickles, chips, frozen dinners—salt is added. In addition, your body conserves sodium during pregnancy and is less likely to excrete it.

The mild swelling that occurs in your body or just in your extremities toward the end of pregnancy has little to do with the amount of salt you eat. Restricting salt severely in an effort to reduce this problem may actually make the swelling worse and aggravate pregnancy-induced high blood pressure. (See "Trouble Spots—Pregnancy-induced Hypertension," Month 5, and "Swelling," Month 9, for more information.)

Using moderate amounts of salt throughout pregnancy is probably the most healthful approach. Empty the salt shaker and reduce the amount of salt you add to homemade foods. Use fresh fruits, juices, baldy pretzels, and lightly salted popcorn instead of salty chips and nuts. If you rely on frozen or take-out meals, buy entrées only, not complete dinners, and serve the main dish with a fresh salad or vegetables to hold down the amount of salt in the meal.

GIVE SOME THOUGHT TO USING ARTIFICIAL SWEETENERS

Three artificial sweeteners have been approved by the FDA for use as an ingredient in food or as a tabletop sweetener: saccharin, aspartame, and acesulfame-K.

Sweet Substitutes

Chemical Name	Ingredient Trade Name	Tabletop Sweetener Trade Name
saccharin	saccharin	saccharin
aspartame	NutraSweet	Equal
acesulfame-K	Sunette	Sweet One

Saccharin, available in the United States since 1901, is 300 times sweeter than sugar. It is absorbed very slowly by the body, not broken down and quickly excreted by the kidneys. In the late 1970s saccharin was believed to be a cancer-causing substance, but newer research has cast doubt on these findings. Currently all foods containing saccharin must carry a warning label until further research is completed. The Council on Scientific Affairs of the American Medical Association has recommended limited use of saccharin by pregnant women and young children.

Aspartame, discovered in the mid-1960s, is made up of two protein fragments (amino acids). It is 200 times sweeter than sugar. All the research available shows that aspartame is safe to use during pregnancy. When aspartame is broken down, the by-products are the same as those found in fruits and not unusual for the body to handle.

A very small percentage of women have a rare inborn error known as PKU (phenylketonuria). These individuals cannot handle one of the protein fragments, phenylalanine, found in aspartame and other common foods. For this reason, all foods with aspartame carry a label declaration to alert affected people.

Acesulfame-K was approved by the FDA in 1988 with no exception for use during pregnancy.

The best advice: *Remember—it takes 55,000 calories to support the growth of a full-term baby. Pregnancy is not the time to cut calories. Using small amounts of aspartame or acesulfame-k is fine; use saccharin only occasionally, if at all.*

**DAILY FOOD GUIDE TO
KEY NUTRIENTS NEEDED
DURING PREGNANCY**

To be sure that you get all the key nutrients you and your developing baby need each day, follow this daily food guide. Each day have:

2 to 3 servings (4 to 6 ounces)	protein-rich foods
4 servings	calcium-rich food
5 servings	fruits and vegetables
5 or more servings	breads, cereals, grains (whole grain and enriched varieties)

TRACKING KEY NUTRIENTS ON THE
PREGNANCY FOOD CHECKLIST

1. Record a sample day during each week of pregnancy.
2. Calculate the amount of each key nutrient eaten that day.
3. If you fall short of any of the key nutrients, change your food choices to be sure you've included all the key nutrients you and your developing baby need.

PREGNANCY FOOD CHECKLIST
Month 6, Week 1

	CAL	PRO (G)	VIT C (MG)	FOL (MCG)	CA (MG)	IR (MG)
BREAKFAST:						
Subtotal	——	——	——	——	——	——
SNACK:						
Subtotal	——	——	——	——	——	——
LUNCH:						
Subtotal	——	——	——	——	——	——
SNACK:						
Subtotal	——	——	——	——	——	——
DINNER:						
Subtotal	——	——	——	——	——	——
SNACK:						
Subtotal	——	——	——	——	——	——
Daily Totals	——	——	——	——	——	——
Daily Nutrient Goals	2200	60	70	400	1200	30

PREGNANCY FOOD CHECKLIST
Month 6, Week 2

	CAL	PRO (G)	VIT C (MG)	FOL (MCG)	CA (MG)	IR (MG)
BREAKFAST:						
Subtotal	—	—	—	—	—	—
SNACK:						
Subtotal	—	—	—	—	—	—
LUNCH:						
Subtotal	—	—	—	—	—	—
SNACK:						
Subtotal	—	—	—	—	—	—
DINNER:						
Subtotal	—	—	—	—	—	—
SNACK:						
Subtotal	—	—	—	—	—	—
Daily Totals	—	—	—	—	—	—
Daily Nutrient Goals	2200	60	70	400	1200	30

PREGNANCY FOOD CHECKLIST
Month 6, Week 3

	CAL	PRO (G)	VIT C (MG)	FOL (MCG)	CA (MG)	IR (MG)
BREAKFAST:						
Subtotal	—	—	—	—	—	—
SNACK:						
Subtotal	—	—	—	—	—	—
LUNCH:						
Subtotal	—	—	—	—	—	—
SNACK:						
Subtotal	—	—	—	—	—	—
DINNER:						
Subtotal	—	—	—	—	—	—
SNACK:						
Subtotal	—	—	—	—	—	—
Daily Totals	—	—	—	—	—	—
Daily Nutrient Goals	2200	60	70	400	1200	30

PREGNANCY FOOD CHECKLIST
Month 6, Week 4

	CAL	PRO (G)	VIT C (MG)	FOL (MCG)	CA (MG)	IR (MG)
BREAKFAST:						
Subtotal	—	—	—	—	—	—
SNACK:						
Subtotal	—	—	—	—	—	—
LUNCH:						
Subtotal	—	—	—	—	—	—
SNACK:						
Subtotal	—	—	—	—	—	—
DINNER:						
Subtotal	—	—	—	—	—	—
SNACK:						
Subtotal	—	—	—	—	—	—
Daily Totals	—	—	—	—	—	—
Daily Nutrient Goals	2200	60	70	400	1200	30

MONTH 6

Month _____   Year _____

Your feelings:

_____
_____
_____
_____
_____
_____

Your questions for your doctor or nurse-midwife:

_____
_____
_____
_____
_____
_____
_____
_____
_____
_____
_____

THE

THIRD

TRIMESTER

MONTH 7

A Mother's Journal

WEEK 25

WEEK 26

During my examination, the doctor felt my abdomen and said the baby weighed between 2 and 2½ pounds. I don't know how the doctor knew that just by feeling my stomach, but I was thrilled with the news. I drove home trying to feel the area where I thought my baby's head was supposed to be.

WEEK 27

WEEK 28

Tonight we attended our first natural childbirth class. We agreed that I had the smallest belly in the group of ten. When we got home, I noticed a slight brownish discharge. I assumed something was very wrong and called my doctor, who assured me that this sometimes happens when the cervix begins to thin out. The doctor said it should end in a couple of days. The discharge lasted a week. Except for this very disturbing episode, I've had an uneventful pregnancy . . . so far.

YOUR BABY

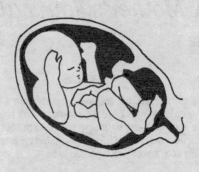

At the end of this month your baby will be two-thirds grown, weighing almost 3 pounds. Although your baby can now swallow, taste, hear, and regulate its body temperature, he still depends on your support to continue to grow. He is getting bigger and stronger with each passing day.

YOUR BODY

As you enter the final three months of pregnancy—the last trimester—you're feeling a little uncomfortable. You are tired of waiting and eager for your baby's arrival. At the same time you feel relieved. The frequent movements are a reassuring sign of your baby's health. The chance of an early miscarriage is over, and every passing day brings you closer to your due date. You're on the homestretch!

Your baby is beginning his last growth spurt before birth. You're aware something is going on because while everyone else is freezing you are dying of the heat! It takes a lot of energy to help your baby develop into a healthy full-term infant. That's why in the last trimester your basal metabolic rate—the rate at which calories are burned for energy when the body is at rest—increases. This increase helps to meet your baby's demands for growth in the last few months, gives you a spurt of energy to get you through the final sprint before delivery, makes you less tolerant to heat, and reduces your ability to get a prolonged, restful night's sleep.

As your baby's size increases daily, your abdominal cavity is pushed up and packed against your diaphragm. This pressure prevents the diaphragm from expanding normally, and you feel breathless. Sometime within the next six to eight weeks your baby will drop lower down into your pelvis. This can happen quickly or slowly, taking a couple of weeks. When it happens, you'll be able to breathe easier and you'll feel less pressure on your stomach. But what is no longer up is now down, causing baby's weight to put increasing pressure on your bowel and bladder.

The pressure from the enlarging uterus also pushes your heart up and to the left. This repositioning along with the extra work the heart is already doing to pump your increased blood volume may make your heartbeat more obvious. Some women report their heart is fluttering. A normal heart can easily accommodate itself to this pregnancy-induced stress, so don't be frightened if you experience these changes.

BACK TO THE BATHROOM

As your baby turns head-down and drops farther into the birth canal, you may find you experience constipation. Because of their greatly enlarged shape, some women find they cannot even sit comfortably to expel a bowel movement. A daily walk to give gravity a boost is one simple way to strengthen muscles and keep bowels regular. Drinking adequate fluids (see Month 3) and increasing the fiber in your diet is also important. Fiber, discussed more fully in the next section, is the part of plants that we cannot digest. It passes through the digestive tract adding bulk and absorbing moisture. The result is softer, larger stools, which are easier to pass. Avoiding constipation often allows you to avoid another complication of late pregnancy—hemorrhoids, an inflammation and protrusion of the hemorrhoidal veins in the rectum.

As your baby turns down, readying for delivery, the bulk of his weight is directly over your bladder, squashing it against the pubic bone and greatly reducing its capacity. This may give you an almost constant urge to urinate. You may even leak a few drops of urine when you laugh or sneeze. Having your baby is the ultimate resolution to this problem! In the meantime, answer the urge to urinate, even if it is only a few drops. Stop drinking fluid two or three hours before bedtime and sleep on your side. This will eliminate some but not all of the nighttime trips to the bathroom.

YOUR DIET: ADDING FIBER

Fiber is important to good health, but most Americans don't get enough of it. Experts recommend 25 to 30 grams of fiber a day—twice as much as the 12 grams most Americans are currently eating.

Fiber is part of many foods we eat. Plant foods like whole grains, beans, lentils, fruit, and vegetables have the most. Meat, fish, poultry, eggs, milk, and cheese have none. Fiber is not considered a nutrient because it isn't digested and absorbed. It simply passes through the digestive tract and does not supply calories.

You may wonder, then, why do you need it? Your digestive tract is one of the largest muscles in your body, and like any muscle, it needs exercise, especially toward the end of pregnancy when it is sandwiched between your growing baby and your backbone. Moving fiber along the intestine exercises the muscle.

Even if you have never been constipated before, you may have this problem during pregnancy. Eating more fiber will relieve constipation and the symptoms of hemorrhoids.

It's easy to make high fiber choices. A high fiber breakfast cereal, one that has two or more grams of fiber in a serving, along with some fresh or dried fruit is a good way to start the day. Eat your breakfast fruit rather than drinking it.

At lunch reach for whole grain breads for sandwiches and whole grain crackers to go with soup. Bean and lentil soups are good choices. Enjoy unpeeled or dried fruits for dessert.

At dinner add some chickpeas and whole wheat croutons to your salad. Don't leave the potato skin on your plate; make a point of eating this fiber-rich part. Enjoy blueberry cobbler or a baked apple for dessert; both are fiber-rich treats.

In the kitchen:

- When a recipe calls for white flour, substitute one-half whole wheat flour and one-half regular flour.
- Use wheat bran in place of some of the bread crumbs in breading or topping.
- Add beans to soup, stews, and salads.
- Keep chunks of unpeeled vegetables in the refrigerator for snacking.

FOR A FIBER BOOST

INSTEAD OF:	TRY:
White bread	Whole wheat bread
Pasta	Whole wheat pasta
White rice	Brown rice
Fruit juice	Whole fruits
Vegetable juice	Whole vegetables
Peeled potatoes	Unpeeled potatoes
Farina	Oatmeal
Puffed rice	Raisin bran
English muffin	Whole grain English muffin
Pretzels	Whole wheat pretzels
Sugar cookies	Fig cookies
Jelly	Whole berry jam

GIVE SOME THOUGHT TO: SUGAR

Each of us eats about 120 pounds of sugar and other sweeteners each year. And that may be the problem—not that sugar is bad for us, but that we eat too much of it instead of picking more nourishing foods. Sugar is a simple carbohydrate that provides about 16 calories in a teaspoon and little else. It is often referred to as an "empty calorie" food—empty of any of the key nutrients.

While you are pregnant, enjoying some sugar on your cereal or a little jelly on your toast is simply a sweet treat and nothing more. If you feel like something sweet, try a handful of presweetened breakfast cereal. It tastes good, is low in fat, and is made from a grain that is rich in B vitamins and fortified with iron—a much more healthful sweet treat than a candy bar or a piece of cake.

The best advice: *Eating too many foods that are high in sugar you may crowd out key nutrients that are more important than ever before for your baby's final growth before birth.*

DAILY FOOD GUIDE TO
KEY NUTRIENTS NEEDED
DURING PREGNANCY

To be sure that you get all the key nutrients you and your developing baby need each day, follow this daily food guide. Each day have:

2 to 3 servings (4 to 6 ounces)	protein-rich foods
4 servings	calcium-rich food
5 servings	fruits and vegetables
5 or more servings	breads, cereals, grains (whole grain and enriched varieties)

TRACKING KEY NUTRIENTS ON THE
PREGNANCY FOOD CHECKLIST

1. Record a sample day during each week of pregnancy.
2. Calculate the amount of each key nutrient eaten that day.
3. If you fall short of any of the key nutrients, change your food choices to be sure you've included all the key nutrients you and your developing baby need.

PREGNANCY FOOD CHECKLIST
Month 7, Week 1

	CAL	PRO (G)	VIT C (MG)	FOL (MCG)	CA (MG)	IR (MG)
BREAKFAST:						
Subtotal	—	—	—	—	—	—
SNACK:						
Subtotal	—	—	—	—	—	—
LUNCH:						
Subtotal	—	—	—	—	—	—
SNACK:						
Subtotal	—	—	—	—	—	—
DINNER:						
Subtotal	—	—	—	—	—	—
SNACK:						
Subtotal	—	—	—	—	—	—
Daily Totals	—	—	—	—	—	—
Daily Nutrient Goals	2200	60	70	400	1200	30

PREGNANCY FOOD CHECKLIST
Month 7, Week 2

	CAL	PRO (G)	VIT C (MG)	FOL (MCG)	CA (MG)	IR (MG)
BREAKFAST:						
Subtotal	——	——	——	——	——	——
SNACK:						
Subtotal	——	——	——	——	——	——
LUNCH:						
Subtotal	——	——	——	——	——	——
SNACK:						
Subtotal	——	——	——	——	——	——
DINNER:						
Subtotal	——	——	——	——	——	——
SNACK:						
Subtotal	——	——	——	——	——	——
Daily Totals	——	——	——	——	——	——
Daily Nutrient Goals	2200	60	70	400	1200	30

PREGNANCY FOOD CHECKLIST
Month 7, Week 3

	CAL	PRO (G)	VIT C (MG)	FOL (MCG)	CA (MG)	IR (MG)
BREAKFAST:						
Subtotal	___	___	___	___	___	___
SNACK:						
Subtotal	___	___	___	___	___	___
LUNCH:						
Subtotal	___	___	___	___	___	___
SNACK:						
Subtotal	___	___	___	___	___	___
DINNER:						
Subtotal	___	___	___	___	___	___
SNACK:						
Subtotal	___	___	___	___	___	___
Daily Totals	___	___	___	___	___	___
Daily Nutrient Goals	2200	60	70	400	1200	30

PREGNANCY FOOD CHECKLIST
Month 7, Week 4

	CAL	PRO (G)	VIT C (MG)	FOL (MCG)	CA (MG)	IR (MG)
BREAKFAST:						
Subtotal	—	—	—	—	—	—
SNACK:						
Subtotal	—	—	—	—	—	—
LUNCH:						
Subtotal	—	—	—	—	—	—
SNACK:						
Subtotal	—	—	—	—	—	—
DINNER:						
Subtotal	—	—	—	—	—	—
SNACK:						
Subtotal	—	—	—	—	—	—
Daily Totals	—	—	—	—	—	—
Daily Nutrient Goals	2200	60	70	400	1200	30

MONTH 7

Month _____ Year _____

Your feelings:

_____

_____

_____

_____

_____

_____

Your questions for your doctor, nurse-midwife, or childbirth educator:

_____

_____

_____

_____

_____

_____

_____

_____

_____

_____

_____

MONTH 8

A Mother's Journal

WEEK 29

The baby hiccups all the time!

WEEK 30

I started getting very annoying cramps in my calves. I've also been experiencing a pulling sensation around the top of my uterus. The doctor said it's normal and is due to the expanding size and weight of the baby. My sides are constantly itchy. Applying skin cream doesn't give me any relief.

WEEK 31

It's difficult to find a comfortable position to sleep. If I lie on my back I feel as if there's a pile of bricks on my chest.

WEEK 32

I gained 7 pounds this month, and I feel like an elephant!

YOUR BABY

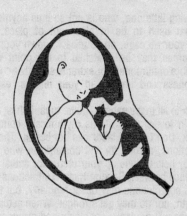

Gone are your baby's days of doing cartwheels. At 4 pounds, 16 inches, your baby now fits more snugly in your uterus, and although still active, his movements feel more like stretching than kicking. Fat deposits are building up under baby's skin, making it smoother. The digestive tract and lungs are almost fully matured, and fine scalp hair is getting longer and thicker.

YOUR BODY

It's 5:00 A.M. and you've already made six trips to the bathroom. All you want is another hour or two of uninterrupted sleep before the alarm rings, when *zap!*—your calf muscle contracts into a triple knot. Here are some suggested remedies: massage the muscle; flex your toes; stand up and put gentle pressure on your leg; or stand on a cold bathroom floor. The enlarging uterus puts pressure on your blood vessels and on the nerves to your legs, which impairs your circulation. This causes the cramping.

So many unusual sensations happen in your body toward the end of pregnancy that you may start to wonder if everything is normal. End-of-pregnancy discomforts are quite normal, and most women experience some if not all of them. Numerous spots on your body begin to ache, puff, itch, swell, hurt, sag, get numb, and feel sore. Fun!

Your growing little one, who is not so little anymore, is pushing everything that used to be in place out of place. The result is pressure—in your rib cage, on your back, down your legs. The skin on your abdomen may be stretched to the point where you will experience spots of numbness or extreme sensitivity. It's not unusual to feel numbness and tingling in your fingers, especially in the morning.

In addition to all these nagging pulls, tugs, itches, and pressures, you may begin to feel your uterus rhythmically contract, get hard, and then relax. Don't panic; labor has not begun. These are Braxton Hicks contractions, named for the obstetrician who first described them, and they help to tone up your uterus for actual labor. You can tell the difference between Braxton Hicks contractions and real labor. Braxton Hicks contractions may occur regularly, but they do not get longer in length, nor do they get stronger. When actual labor begins, the contractions will gradually get closer and stronger, and they will last longer.

EXCUSE ME, I BURPED!

Gas, indigestion, belching, and heartburn are partly the result of the hormone progesterone and partly the result of the compression of your digestive tract between your growing baby and your backbone. Progesterone causes relaxation of the smooth muscles of your uterus so that it can expand as your baby grows, but this hormone also has a relaxing effect on other smooth muscles in your body, including those in your digestive tract. This relaxation slows down the normal action of the gut, which allows more time for nutrients to be absorbed. But this slowing down can also result in discomfort when contents of the digestive tract are not moved along at a normal rate.

Here are a few tips that will help you feel better. Try eating smaller, more frequent meals rather than three large meals a day. If you eat out in the evening, order two appetizers rather than an appetizer and a main dish, to keep portions smaller. Steer clear of fried and fatty foods. Concentrate on carbohydrates instead—stir-fried and pasta dishes are good choices, but skip the cream sauce. And don't eat right before bedtime.

If you are bothered by embarrassing gas, eat slowly with your mouth closed, sip beverages through a straw, and don't chew gum, which increases the amount of air you swallow and makes the problem worse. Foods that cause gas in one person may not in another. Beans have a reputation for causing gas, but other foods can be culprits, too: onions, celery, cabbage, cauliflower, cucumbers, bananas, prune juice, bagels, and even applesauce. Foods with a lot of incorporated air, like whipped cream and carbonated beverages, can increase gas and cause belching. You'll need to determine for yourself which foods are giving you the most trouble; then simply eat fewer of those items or cut them out completely for the next few weeks.

YOUR DIET: FAT AND CHOLESTEROL

Everywhere you turn, you hear or read that high levels of fat and cholesterol in the blood can lead to heart attack and stroke. You know that too much fat and cholesterol are not good, but you are not sure how much you should cut down while you are pregnant.

Most experts agree that adults should get 30 percent of their daily calories from fat and eat no more than 300 milligrams of cholesterol each day. This is good advice during pregnancy, too. Cutting back dramatically on fat or cholesterol during pregnancy is not wise. Fat calories provide more than twice the energy (9 calories per gram) of protein and carbohydrate calories (both of which supply 4 calories per gram).

Remember, it takes 55,000 calories to support the full-term growth of your developing baby, so a concentrated source of calories—a little fat each day—is beneficial. Lean meat, fish, and poultry; low-fat milk, cheese, and yogurt; and a dessert now and then are good sources of needed fat calories.

Most people think of cholesterol as a harmful substance that clogs the arteries and increases the risk for heart disease. You might be surprised to find out that cholesterol is in every cell of your body and your baby's and is essential for proper development. You get cholesterol in two ways: you absorb it from food, and you make it in your liver. When the level of cholesterol in your blood gets too high, it can cause trouble. That is why the National Cholesterol Education Program has recommended that people over the age of twenty have their cholesterol tested at least once every five years. Health agencies often set up convenient screening sites in supermarkets, at malls, and in community clinics. Fathers-to-be should take advantage of this service. *Pregnant women should not have their cholesterol tested.*

When you are pregnant your blood fat levels change. Total cholesterol, triglycerides, and LDL and VLDL cholesterol go up and then level off shortly before your baby is born. If you have your cholesterol screened now, you may become alarmed by these higher-than-normal levels. Values will return to prepregnancy levels within a few months after your baby is born.

Foods that are high in fat are usually high in cholesterol as well. If you are eating moderate amounts of fat, you are probably eating moderate amounts of cholesterol, too. This is fine for the time being.

Because so many foods in the supermarket are labeled "low cholesterol" or "cholesterol free," you might be confused about which foods actually have cholesterol and which don't. It is easy to determine the difference if you remember one simple rule: *Foods that have feet, fins, wings, or claws contain cholesterol; foods that grow in the ground do not.*

To apply this rule think about a few foods that contain fat: corn oil, butter, hamburger, milk, and peanuts. Corn oil and peanuts grow in the ground, so even though they have fat, they do not have cholesterol. Hamburger comes from a steer and milk and butter come from a cow, both of which have feet, so these foods not only have fat, they also have cholesterol.

Now you can no longer be fooled by labels that are somewhat misleading—such as a peanut butter jar that touts itself as "cholesterol free." Peanuts grow in the ground, so they've never had cholesterol. This means that every brand of peanut butter on the shelf is cholesterol free whether its label says so or not. As more and more new products appear in the supermarket it is important for you to know how to pick the best ones for yourself and your family.

FAT FACTS

Cholesterol: A fatlike substance in every cell in the body; found in animal foods.

HDL cholesterol: "Good" cholesterol which carries the type of cholesterol that is broken down and removed from the body.

VLDL and LDL cholesterol: "Bad" cholesterol which carries the type of cholesterol that is deposited in the arteries.

Fat: A concentrated source of energy (calories); eat moderate amounts.

Saturated fat: Fat that is solid at room temperature; found mainly in animal foods.

Polyunsaturated fat: Fat that is liquid at room temperature; found mainly in plant foods.

Monounsaturated fat: Fat that becomes partly solid when chilled; found in olive oil, peanuts, soybean oil, and canola oil.

Use moderate amounts of all fats for good health.

GIVE SOME THOUGHT TO: MEAL SKIPPING

Your baby's growth is continuous and rapid at this point, requiring a steady supply of nutrients. When you skip a meal, ask yourself, "Who's feeding my baby?"

At the end of pregnancy, going without food for a prolonged period of time is not wise. Research has shown that when pregnant women fast, even for a period as short as one day, they increase their risk of spontaneous premature labor and delivery.

The best advice: *Continue to eat regularly and make good food choices. You want to give your baby all the nutrients she needs to get ready to face the world in the best possible health.*

DAILY FOOD GUIDE TO
KEY NUTRIENTS NEEDED
DURING PREGNANCY

To be sure that you get all the key nutrients you and your developing baby need each day, follow this daily food guide. Each day have:

2 to 3 servings (4 to 6 ounces)	protein-rich foods
4 servings	calcium-rich food
5 servings	fruits and vegetables
5 or more servings	breads, cereals, grains (whole grain and enriched varieties)

TRACKING KEY NUTRIENTS ON THE
PREGNANCY FOOD CHECKLIST

1. Record a sample day during each week of pregnancy.
2. Calculate the amount of each key nutrient eaten that day.
3. If you fall short of any of the key nutrients, change your food choices to be sure you've included all the key nutrients you and your developing baby need.

PREGNANCY FOOD CHECKLIST
Month 8, Week 1

	CAL	PRO (G)	VIT C (MG)	FOL (MCG)	CA (MG)	IR (MG)
BREAKFAST:						
Subtotal	—	—	—	—	—	—
SNACK:						
Subtotal	—	—	—	—	—	—
LUNCH:						
Subtotal	—	—	—	—	—	—
SNACK:						
Subtotal	—	—	—	—	—	—
DINNER:						
Subtotal	—	—	—	—	—	—
SNACK:						
Subtotal	—	—	—	—	—	—
Daily Totals	—	—	—	—	—	—
Daily Nutrient Goals	2200	60	70	400	1200	30

PREGNANCY FOOD CHECKLIST
Month 8, Week 2

	CAL	PRO (G)	VIT C (MG)	FOL (MCG)	CA (MG)	IR (MG)
BREAKFAST:						
Subtotal	—	—	—	—	—	—
SNACK:						
Subtotal	—	—	—	—	—	—
LUNCH:						
Subtotal	—	—	—	—	—	—
SNACK:						
Subtotal	—	—	—	—	—	—
DINNER:						
Subtotal	—	—	—	—	—	—
SNACK:						
Subtotal	—	—	—	—	—	—
Daily Totals	—	—	—	—	—	—
Daily Nutrient Goals	2200	60	70	400	1200	30

PREGNANCY FOOD CHECKLIST
Month 8, Week 3

	CAL	PRO (G)	VIT C (MG)	FOL (MCG)	CA (MG)	IR (MG)
BREAKFAST:						
Subtotal	—	—	—	—	—	—
SNACK:						
Subtotal	—	—	—	—	—	—
LUNCH:						
Subtotal	—	—	—	—	—	—
SNACK:						
Subtotal	—	—	—	—	—	—
DINNER:						
Subtotal	—	—	—	—	—	—
SNACK:						
Subtotal	—	—	—	—	—	—
Daily Totals	—	—	—	—	—	—
Daily Nutrient Goals	2200	60	70	400	1200	30

PREGNANCY FOOD CHECKLIST
Month 8, Week 4

	CAL	PRO (G)	VIT C (MG)	FOL (MCG)	CA (MG)	IR (MG)
BREAKFAST:						
Subtotal	——	——	——	——	——	——
SNACK:						
Subtotal	——	——	——	——	——	——
LUNCH:						
Subtotal	——	——	——	——	——	——
SNACK:						
Subtotal	——	——	——	——	——	——
DINNER:						
Subtotal	——	——	——	——	——	——
SNACK:						
Subtotal	——	——	——	——	——	——
Daily Totals	——	——	——	——	——	——
Daily Nutrient Goals	2200	60	70	400	1200	30

MONTH 8

Month _____ Year _____

Your feelings:

_____
_____
_____
_____
_____
_____

Your questions for your doctor, nurse-midwife, or childbirth educator:

_____
_____
_____
_____
_____
_____
_____
_____
_____
_____
_____

MONTH 9

A Mother's Journal

WEEK 33

The baby kicks so much at night that I have trouble sleeping.

WEEK 34

As my due date approaches, I'm apprehensive about the delivery. My biggest fear is that I won't be able to reach my husband.

WEEK 35

The dark line down the middle of my abdomen is expanding. At this rate it should extend up to my nose by next week! I continue to practice Lamaze exercises. I'm beginning to wonder if they will help.

WEEK 36

I'm so large I have to roll over on my side to get out of bed. I feel like a blimp!

TILL DELIVERY

I'm five days past my due date, so I was scheduled for a fetal nonstress test. It was a simple procedure. I was told to lie on my back, and a belt attached to a monitor was wrapped around my stomach to monitor the bay. The test showed that everything is fine.

Five days later George was born at 21½ inches, weighing 7 pounds 14 ounces.

YOUR BABY

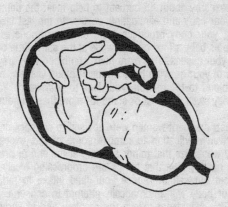

By the end of this month your baby is fully grown, weighing 7 to 7½ pounds and about 20 inches long. Your baby's eyes are blue, but they may change color shortly after birth. The fine downy body hair is disappearing, fingernails are hard, tooth buds are in place, and lungs are ready for their first cry.

Your baby is ready to be on his own. It won't be long now!

YOUR BODY

Over the last nine months you have nurtured a single microscopic cell into a six thousand billion–celled human being. In a few short weeks your baby will be born.

Your baby is probably in a head-down position at the entrance of the birth canal. Growth has continued to the point where he fits snugly in your enlarged uterus and can't move around as freely. It's normal for your baby to become less active as the ninth month progresses.

SWELLING

Over 50 percent of all pregnant women experience some puffiness in their ankles. During pregnancy the fluid volume of your bloodstream increases by about 45 percent to help meet the demands of nourishing your baby and eliminating wastes. In the last few weeks before labor, your body produces more of the hormone estrogen, which promotes baby's final growth while at the same time conserving fluids in your tissues. This extra fluid, combined with gravity and the pressure of your growing baby on major blood vessels, makes it difficult for blood to return from your legs to your heart. Your feet and ankles may swell if you sit or stand for more than an hour in one place.

In the past, pregnant women were advised to cut back on salt or they were given medication to remove some of this excess body water. Today we realize that minor swelling at the end of pregnancy is actually a healthy sign that things are progressing nicely. If you attempt to cut out salt or reduce your fluid intake to reduce the swelling, your body will automatically attempt to conserve sodium and water. This would not relieve the problem and in some cases might make it worse by causing blood pressure to rise.

To reduce swelling or prevent the problem before it begins, you should exercise regularly. Walking, swimming, cycling, and even rocking in a rocking chair all stimulate blood flow from the legs to the heart. Elevate your feet regularly throughout the day. Lying down and raising your legs above the level of your heart, for even a few minutes, is very beneficial. Avoid clothes, shoes, and knee socks that are tight. Don't sit with your legs crossed. At night sleep on your left side.

LABOR

A number of signs will appear shortly to alert you to the beginning of labor. Pressure will ease on your diaphragm and stomach as your baby settles lower into your pelvis. A blood-streaked discharge may occur if the mucous plug at the mouth of the uterus dislodges. The amniotic sac (baby-cushioning water bag) may crack and leak clear fluid or it may break and release two to three cups of fluid at one time. Keep your doctor informed as these events happen.

If you think you are in labor, eat nothing and drink fluids sparingly.

The beginning of labor is actually the end of a whole series of events. The uterus has stretched to its limits. The placenta ages, decreasing its production of the hormone progesterone (the pregnancy-holding hormone) and reducing its ability to deliver nutrients and oxygen and remove wastes from your developing baby. The level of the hormone oxytocinase decreases, allowing the level of a second hormone, oxytocin, to increase. Oxytocin makes the uterus contract during labor. There is increasing evidence that your baby may actually be the final trigger that starts labor.

There are three stages of labor:

1. First stage—from the first labor contraction until the cervix (mouth of the uterus) is fully dilated (10 centimeters). If it hasn't happened already, the mucous plug will release and the amniotic sac will break. This stage lasts about ten to twelve hours in first-time mothers and seven or less in subsequent pregnancies.
2. Second stage—begins when the cervix is completely dilated and ends with the delivery of your baby. This stage lasts from thirty to ninety minutes for first-time mothers and can be twenty minutes or less in subsequent pregnancies.
3. Third stage—begins with the birth of your baby and ends with the delivery of the placenta (afterbirth). It lasts from five to twenty-five minutes.

OVERDUE?

Only one in twenty women delivers on her due date. In a normal pregnancy, labor may begin up to two weeks before or two weeks after the calculated due date. You're not overdue until you are at least two weeks beyond your expected date of delivery.

YOUR DIET: FEEDING BABY

As delivery draws near, you are probably less worried about what you are eating and more concerned with what you are going to feed your baby. Over the next year you will be making many decisions about how, what, and when to feed your baby.

Today more and more new mothers are choosing to breast-feed

their babies. What should you decide? Breast-feeding seems natural, and everyone is doing it. You feel guilty thinking about bottle-feeding your new baby, but you may need to return to work soon. You've never seen a baby nursed and are not sure you could do it. You may even feel a little uncomfortable about the intimacy of breast-feeding and unsure how you would handle it. You may also be nervous that you will not know how to prepare formula correctly.

All of these concerns are normal. Very few new mothers decide to nurse or bottle-feed without a few moments of doubt about the decision they have made. Take time and learn about both. This, like many things you will decide for your baby, has no right or wrong answer. The decision you make should be one that you feel comfortable with. If you do, then you've made the right choice.

BREAST AND BOTTLE BASICS

- Nursing is a natural process; you can be successful at it if you have some knowledge and some patience.
- Breast milk is the most ideal food for a newborn infant.
- Infant formula is the best alternative to breast milk.
- Breast-feeding or bottle-feeding, or combining the two, provides your baby with excellent nutrition.

There is no hard and fast rule about when to begin your baby on solid food. It is almost easier to tell you when *not* to give it. Newborns do not need food, and very few babies should be given food before they are four months of age. Even then they need very little.

You can begin introducing a few simple foods sometime during the fourth month. But before you do, be sure your baby is showing signs of readiness. Can he swallow as well as suck? Can he sit by himself with support? Can he control the movement of his head and neck? Is he showing interest in eating?

Once you feel comfortable that your baby is ready for food, when he or she is at least four months old, you need only remember these three easy steps:

1. Feed simple foods.
2. Give small amounts.
3. Introduce no more than one new food a week.

FEEDING YOUR BABY

MONTH	FOOD
1, 2, 3	Breast milk or Infant formula
4, 5	Single grain cereals, Banana, Applesauce
6	Other simple fruits, Simple vegetables
7	Cereal combinations, Fruit combinations, Juice, Egg yolk
8	Combination vegetables, Meat, Poultry, Fish, Whole eggs
9, 10	Combination dinners, Beans, Cheese, Yogurt
11, 12	Finger foods, Dry cereal

This chart is not meant to be followed rigidly. It is simply a guide to your baby's readiness for various solid foods.

GIVE SOME THOUGHT TO THE FUTURE

You've spent the last nine months taking good care of yourself— eating well, exercising, and getting plenty of rest. You've learned a lot about nutrition, and you've incorporated these principles into your everyday eating habits.

Now it's your turn to be the teacher—teaching your newborn child good health habits.

The best advice: *What you do right now will affect your health twenty years from now. Continue to take good care of yourself.*

DAILY FOOD GUIDE TO
KEY NUTRIENTS NEEDED
DURING PREGNANCY

To be sure that you get all the key nutrients you and your developing baby need each day, follow this daily food guide. Each day have:

2 to 3 servings (4 to 6 ounces)	protein-rich foods
4 servings	calcium-rich food
5 servings	fruits and vegetables
5 or more servings	breads, cereals, grains (whole grain and enriched varieties)

TRACKING KEY NUTRIENTS ON THE
PREGNANCY FOOD CHECKLIST

1. Record a sample day during each week of pregnancy.
2. Calculate the amount of each key nutrient eaten that day.
3. If you fall short of any of the key nutrients, change your food choices to be sure you've included all the key nutrients you and your developing baby need.

PREGNANCY FOOD CHECKLIST
Month 9, Week 1

	CAL	PRO (G)	VIT C (MG)	FOL (MCG)	CA (MG)	IR (MG)
BREAKFAST:						
Subtotal	___	___	___	___	___	___
SNACK:						
Subtotal	___	___	___	___	___	___
LUNCH:						
Subtotal	___	___	___	___	___	___
SNACK:						
Subtotal	___	___	___	___	___	___
DINNER:						
Subtotal	___	___	___	___	___	___
SNACK:						
Subtotal	___	___	___	___	___	___
Daily Totals	___	___	___	___	___	___
Daily Nutrient Goals	2200	60	70	400	1200	30

PREGNANCY FOOD CHECKLIST
Month 9, Week 2

	CAL	PRO (G)	VIT C (MG)	FOL (MCG)	CA (MG)	IR (MG)
BREAKFAST:						
Subtotal	—	—	—	—	—	—
SNACK:						
Subtotal	—	—	—	—	—	—
LUNCH:						
Subtotal	—	—	—	—	—	—
SNACK:						
Subtotal	—	—	—	—	—	—
DINNER:						
Subtotal	—	—	—	—	—	—
SNACK:						
Subtotal	—	—	—	—	—	—
Daily Totals	—	—	—	—	—	—
Daily Nutrient Goals	2200	60	70	400	1200	30

PREGNANCY FOOD CHECKLIST
Month 9, Week 3

	CAL	PRO (G)	VIT C (MG)	FOL (MCG)	CA (MG)	IR (MG)
BREAKFAST:						
Subtotal	—	—	—	—	—	—
SNACK:						
Subtotal	—	—	—	—	—	—
LUNCH:						
Subtotal	—	—	—	—	—	—
SNACK:						
Subtotal	—	—	—	—	—	—
DINNER:						
Subtotal	—	—	—	—	—	—
SNACK:						
Subtotal	—	—	—	—	—	—
Daily Totals	—	—	—	—	—	—
Daily Nutrient Goals	2200	60	70	400	1200	30

PREGNANCY FOOD CHECKLIST
Month 9, Week 4

	CAL	PRO (G)	VIT C (MG)	FOL (MCG)	CA (MG)	IR (MG)
BREAKFAST:						
Subtotal	——	——	——	——	——	——
SNACK:						
Subtotal	——	——	——	——	——	——
LUNCH:						
Subtotal	——	——	——	——	——	——
SNACK:						
Subtotal	——	——	——	——	——	——
DINNER:						
Subtotal	——	——	——	——	——	——
SNACK:						
Subtotal	——	——	——	——	——	——
Daily Totals	——	——	——	——	——	——
Daily Nutrient Goals	2200	60	70	400	1200	30

<u>MONTH 9</u>

Month _____ Year _____

Your feelings:

_____
_____
_____
_____
_____
_____

Your questions for your doctor, nurse-midwife, or childbirth educator:

_____
_____
_____
_____
_____
_____
_____
_____
_____
_____
_____

THE
PREGNANCY
NUTRITION
COUNTER

DEFINITIONS

as prep (as prepared): refers to food that has been prepared according to package directions

cooked: refers to food cooked without the addition of fat (oil, butter, margarine, etc.); steaming, broiling, and dry roasting are examples of this type of preparation

home recipe: describes homemade dishes; those included can be used as a guide to the nutrient values of similar dishes

take-out: describes restaurant menu items and ready-to-use products

tr (trace): value used when a food contains less than one calorie, less than one gram of protein, less than one milligram of vitamin C, calcium, or iron, and less than one microgram of folic acid

0" trim: refers to all visible fat removed from outer edge of meat

¼" trim: refers to visible fat trimmed to within ¼ inch of meat.

EQUIVALENT MEASURES

1 tablespoon	=	3 teaspoons
4 tablespoons	=	¼ cup
8 tablespoons	=	½ cup
12 tablespoons	=	¾ cup
16 tablespoons	=	1 cup
28 grams	=	1 ounce

DRY MEASUREMENTS

16 ounces	=	1 pound
12 ounces	=	¾ pound
8 ounces	=	½ pound
4 ounces	=	¼ pound

LIQUID MEASUREMENTS

2 tablespoons	=	1 ounce
¼ cup	=	2 ounces
½ cup	=	4 ounces
¾ cup	=	6 ounces
1 cup	=	8 ounces
2 cups	=	16 ounces
2 cups	=	1 pint
4 cups	=	32 ounces
4 cups	=	1 quart

ABBREVIATIONS

ca	=	calcium	pro	=	protein
cal	=	calories	qt	=	quart
diam	=	diameter	reg	=	regular
fol	=	folic acid	sm	=	small
frzn	=	frozen	sq	=	square
g	=	gram	tbsp	=	tablespoon
ir	=	iron	tr	=	trace
lb	=	pound	tsp	=	teaspoon
lg	=	large	vit C	=	vitamin C
med	=	medium	w/	=	with
oz	=	ounce	w/o	=	without
pkg	=	package	"	=	inch
prep	=	prepared			

Protein values are given in grams.
Vitamin C, calcium, and iron values are given in milligrams.
Folic acid values are given in micrograms.
– indicates no value is available.

FOOD	PORTION	CAL	PRO	VIT C	FOL	CA	IR
ABALONE							
FRESH							
fried	3 oz	161	17	–	5	32	3
raw	3 oz	89	15	–	4	27	3
ACEROLA							
acerola	1 fruit	2	tr	81	–	1	tr
JUICE							
acerola	1 cup	51	1	1232	–	24	1
ADZUKI BEANS							
CANNED							
sweetened	1 cup	702	11	–	–	66	3
DRIED							
cooked	1 cup	294	17	0	–	63	5
raw	1 cup	649	39	0	–	130	10
READY-TO-USE							
yokan; sliced	3¼" slice	112	1	–	–	12	1
AKEE							
fresh	3½ oz	223	5	26	–	40	3
ALFALFA							
sprouts	1 cup	40	1	3	12	10	tr
sprouts	1 tbsp	1	tr	tr	1	1	tr
ALLSPICE							
ground	1 tsp	5	tr	1	–	13	tr
ALMONDS							
almond butter w/o salt	1 tbsp	101	2	tr	10	43	1
almond butter, honey & cinnamon	1 tbsp	96	3	tr	10	43	1
almond meal	1 oz	116	11	–	–	120	2

FOOD	PORTION	CAL	PRO	VIT C	FOL	CA	IR
almond paste	1 oz	127	3	tr	16	65	1
dried, unblanched	1 oz	167	6	tr	16	75	1
dried, blanched	1 oz	166	6	tr	11	70	1
dry roasted, unblanched	1 oz	167	5	tr	18	80	1
dry roasted, unblanched, salted	1 oz	167	5	tr	18	80	1
oil roasted, blanched	1 oz	174	6	tr	18	55	2
oil roasted, blanched, salted	1 oz	174	5	tr	18	55	2
oil roasted, unblanched	1 oz	176	6	tr	18	66	1
toasted, unblanched	1 oz	167	6	tr	18	80	1

AMARANTH

cooked	½ cup	59	1	27	–	138	1
uncooked	½ cup	366	14	4	48	150	7

ANCHOVY

CANNED
in oil	5	42	6	–	–	46	1
in oil	1 can (1.6 oz)	95	13	–	–	104	2

FRESH
raw	3 oz	62	17	–	–	125	3

ANGLERFISH

raw	3½ oz	72	15	–	–	–	–

ANISE

seed	1 tsp	7	tr	–	–	14	1

ANTELOPE

raw	1 oz	32	6	–	–	1	1
roasted	3 oz	127	25	–	–	4	3.6

FOOD	PORTION	CAL	PRO	VIT C	FOL	CA	IR
APPLE							
CANNED							
applesauce, sweetened	½ cup	97	tr	2	1	5	tr
applesauce, unsweetened	½ cup	53	tr	2	1	4	tr
sliced, sweetened	1 cup	136	tr	1	1	4	tr
DRIED							
cooked w/ sugar	½ cup	116	tr	1	–	4	tr
cooked w/o sugar	½ cup	72	tr	1	0	4	tr
rings	10	155	1	3	–	9	1
FRESH							
apple	1	81	tr	8	4	10	tr
w/o skin; sliced	1 cup	62	tr	4	tr	4	tr
w/o skin; sliced & microwaved	1 cup	96	tr	tr	1	8	tr
w/o skin; sliced & cooked	1 cup	91	tr	tr	1	8	tr
FROZEN							
sliced, w/o sugar	½ cup	41	tr	tr	1	4	tr
JUICE							
apple	1 cup	116	tr	2	tr	16	1
frzn; as prep	1 cup	111	tr	1	1	14	1
frzn; not prep	6 oz	349	1	4	2	43	2
APRICOTS							
CANNED							
heavy syrup w/ skin	3 halves	70	tr	3	1	7	tr
juice pack w/ skin	3 halves	40	1	4	–	10	tr
light syrup w/ skin	3 halves	54	tr	2	1	10	tr
water pack w/ skin	3 halves	22	1	3	2	7	tr
water pack w/o skin	4 halves	20	1	2	2	8	tr
DRIED							
halves	10	83	1	1	3	16	2
halves; cooked w/o sugar	½ c	106	2	2	0	20	2

FOOD	PORTION	CAL	PRO	VIT C	FOL	CA	IR
FRESH apricots	3	51	1	11	9	15	1
FROZEN sweetened	½ cup	119	1	11	–	12	1
JUICE nectar	1 cup	141	1	1	3	17	1

ARROWHEAD

FOOD	PORTION	CAL	PRO	VIT C	FOL	CA	IR
fresh; boiled	1 med (⅓ oz)	9	1	–	–	1	tr

ARROWROOT

FOOD	PORTION	CAL	PRO	VIT C	FOL	CA	IR
flour	1 cup	457	tr	0	9	51	tr

ARTICHOKE

FOOD	PORTION	CAL	PRO	VIT C	FOL	CA	IR
FRESH boiled	1 med	53	3	9	61	47	2
hearts; cooked	½ cup	37	2	6	42	33	1
jerusalem, raw; sliced	½ cup	57	2	3	–	10	3
FROZEN cooked	1 pkg (9 oz)	108	7	12	285	50	1

ASPARAGUS

FOOD	PORTION	CAL	PRO	VIT C	FOL	CA	IR
CANNED spears	½ cup	24	3	–	116	–	2
FRESH cooked	½ cup	22	2	18	132	22	1
cooked	4 spears	15	2	16	88	15	tr
raw	½ cup	15	2	22	86	14	tr
FROZEN cooked	4 spears	17	2	15	81	14	tr
cooked	1 pkg (10 oz)	82	9	72	395	68	2

FOOD	PORTION	CAL	PRO	VIT C	FOL	CA	IR
AVOCADO							
FRESH							
avocado	1	324	4	16	124	22	2
puree	1 cup	370	5	18	142	25	2
BACON							
breakfast strips, beef; cooked	3 strips (34 g)	153	11	–	–	–	1
cooked	3 strips	109	6	6	1	2	tr
grilled	2 slices (1.7 oz)	86	11	10	2	5	tr
pork	3 slices (2 oz)	378	–	–	–	5	–
BACON SUBSTITUTES							
bacon substitute	1 strip	25	1	0	3	2	tr
BAGEL							
egg	1 (3½" diam)	200	7	0	–	29	2
plain	1 (3½" diam)	200	7	0	–	29	2
BAKING POWDER							
baking powder	1 tsp	5	tr	0	–	58	0
low sodium	1 tsp	5	tr	0	–	207	0
BALSAM-PEAR							
leafy tips, raw	½ cup	7	1	21	–	20	tr
leafy tips; cooked	½ cup	10	1	16	25	12	tr
pods; cooked	½ cup	12	1	21	–	6	tr

FOOD	PORTION	CAL	PRO	VIT C	FOL	CA	IR

BAMBOO SHOOTS

CANNED							
sliced	1 cup	25	2	1	–	10	tr
FRESH							
cooked	½ cup	15	2	0	–	14	tr
raw	½ cup	21	2	3	–	10	tr

BANANA

DRIED							
powder	1 tbsp	21	tr	tr	–	1	tr
FRESH							
banana	1	105	1	10	22	7	tr

BARLEY

pearled, uncooked	½ cup	352	10	0	23	29	3
pearled; cooked	½ cup	97	2	0	13	8	1

BASIL

ground	1 tsp	4	tr	1	–	30	1

BASS

FRESH							
freshwater, raw	3 oz	97	16	–	–	68	1
sea, raw	3 oz	82	16	–	–	9	tr
sea; cooked	3 oz	105	20	–	–	11	tr
striped, raw	3 oz	82	15	–	–	–	–

BAY LEAF

crumbled	1 tsp	2	tr	tr	–	5	tr

BEANS

CANNED							
baked beans w/ beef	½ cup	161	8	2	–	60	2
baked beans w/ franks	½ cup	182	9	3	38	61	2

FOOD	PORTION	CAL	PRO	VIT C	FOL	CA	IR
baked beans w/ pork	½ cup	133	7	3	46	66	2
baked beans w/ pork & sweet sauce	½ cup	140	7	4	47	77	2
baked beans w/ pork & tomato sauce	½ cup	123	7	4	28	70	4
baked beans, plain	½ cup	118	6	–	30	64	tr
baked beans, vegetarian	½ cup	118	6	–	30	64	tr
HOME RECIPE baked beans	½ cup	190	7	1	61	77	3

BEAR

FOOD	PORTION	CAL	PRO	VIT C	FOL	CA	IR
raw	1 oz	46	6	–	–	1	2
simmered	3 oz	220	28	–	–	4	9

BEAVER

FOOD	PORTION	CAL	PRO	VIT C	FOL	CA	IR
raw	1 oz	41	7	1	–	4	2
simmered	3 oz	141	23	2	–	14	7

BEECHNUTS

FOOD	PORTION	CAL	PRO	VIT C	FOL	CA	IR
dried	1 oz	164	2	–	–	0	–

BEEF

FOOD	PORTION	CAL	PRO	VIT C	FOL	CA	IR
CANNED corned beef	1 oz	71	22	0	–	15	2
corned beef	1 slice (21 g)	53	14	0	–	11	1
FRESH bottom round, lean & fat, trim 0", Choice; roasted	3 oz	172	24	0	10	4	3
bottom round, lean & fat, trim 0", Select; braised	3 oz	171	27	0	9	4	3
bottom round, lean & fat, trim 0", Select; roasted	3 oz	150	24	0	11	4	3
bottom round, lean & fat, trim 0", braised	3 oz	193	26	0	9	4	3

FOOD	PORTION	CAL	PRO	VIT C	FOL	CA	IR
bottom round, lean & fat, trim ¼", Choice; braised	3 oz	241	24	0	8	5	3
bottom round, lean & fat, trim ¼", Choice; roasted	3 oz	221	22	0	10	5	2
bottom round, lean & fat, trim ¼", Select; braised	3 oz	220	25	0	8	5	3
bottom round, lean & fat, trim ¼", Select; roasted	3 oz	199	23	0	10	5	2
brisket, flat half, lean & fat, trim 0"; braised	3 oz	183	26	0	7	5	2
brisket, flat half, lean & fat, trim ¼"; braised	3 oz	309	21	0	5	5	2
brisket, point half, lean & fat, trim 0"; braised	3 oz	304	20	0	6	7	2
brisket, point half, lean & fat, trim ¼"; braised	3 oz	343	19	0	5	7	2
brisket, whole, lean & fat, trim 0"; braised	3 oz	247	23	0	6	6	2
brisket, whole, lean & fat, trim ¼", raw	1 oz	88	5	0	2	2	tr
brisket, whole, lean & fat, trim ¼"; braised	3 oz	327	27	0	5	7	2
chuck arm pot roast, lean & fat, trim 0"; braised	3 oz	238	25	0	8	8	3
chuck arm pot roast, lean & fat, trim ¼"; braised	3 oz	282	23	0	8	9	3
chuck blade roast, lean & fat, trim 0"; braised	3 oz	284	23	0	5	11	3
chuck blade roast, lean & fat, trim ¼"; braised	3 oz	293	23	0	5	11	3
corned beef brisket, raw	14 oz	56	4	8	–	2	tr
corned beef brisket; cooked	3 oz	213	15	–	–	7	2
eye of round, lean & fat, trim 0", Choice; roasted	3 oz	153	24	0	6	4	2

FOOD	PORTION	CAL	PRO	VIT C	FOL	CA	IR
eye of round, lean & fat, trim 0", Select; roasted	3 oz	137	24	0	6	4	2
eye of round, lean & fat, trim ¼", Select; roasted	3 oz	184	23	0	6	5	2
eye of round, lean & fat, trim ¼", Choice; roasted	3 oz	205	23	0	6	5	2
eye of round, lean & fat, trim ¼"; raw	1 oz	60	6	0	2	1	tr
flank, lean & fat, trim 0"; braised	3 oz	224	23	0	7	6	3
flank, lean & fat, trim 0"; broiled	3 oz	192	22	0	7	6	2
ground lean; broiled well done	3 oz	238	24	0	9	10	2
ground regular, raw	4 oz	351	19	0	8	10	2
ground regular; broiled medium	3 oz	246	20	0	8	9	2
ground regular; broiled well done	3 oz	248	23	0	9	10	2
ground, extra lean, raw	4 oz	265	21	0	9	7	2
ground, extra lean; broiled medium	3 oz	217	22	0	8	6	2
ground, extra lean; broiled well done	3 oz	225	24	0	9	7	2
ground, extra lean; fried medium	3 oz	216	21	0	7	6	2
ground, extra lean; fried well done	3 oz	224	24	0	9	7	2
ground, lean, raw	4 oz	298	20	0	9	9	2
ground, lean; broiled medium	3 oz	231	21	0	8	9	2
porterhouse steak, lean only, trim ¼", Choice; broiled	3 oz	185	24	0	7	6	3

FOOD	PORTION	CAL	PRO	VIT C	FOL	CA	IR
porterhouse steak, lean & fat, trim ¼", Choice; broiled	3 oz	260	21	0	6	7	2
rib eye small end, lean & fat, trim 0", Choice; broiled	3 oz	261	21	0	6	11	2
rib large end, lean & fat, trim 0"; roasted	3 oz	300	20	0	6	8	2
rib large end, lean & fat, trim ¼"; broiled	3 oz	295	18	0	5	9	2
rib large end, lean & fat, trim ¼"; roasted	3 oz	310	19	0	6	8	2
rib small end, lean & fat, trim 0"; broiled	3 oz	252	21	0	6	11	2
rib small end, lean & fat, trim ¼"; broiled	3 oz	285	20	0	6	11	2
rib small end, lean & fat, trim ¼"; roasted	3 oz	295	19	0	5	11	2
rib whole, lean & fat, trim ¼", Choice; broiled	3 oz	306	19	0	5	10	2
rib whole, lean & fat, trim ¼", Choice; roasted	3 oz	320	19	0	6	9	2
rib whole, lean & fat, trim ¼", Prime; roasted	3 oz	348	19	0	6	10	2
rib whole, lean & fat, trim ¼", Select; broiled	3 oz	274	19	0	5	10	2
rib whole, lean & fat, trim ¼", Select; roasted	3 oz	286	19	0	6	9	2
shank crosscut, lean & fat, trim ¼", Choice; simmered	3 oz	224	26	0	8	25	3
short loin top loin, lean & fat, trim 0", Choice; broiled	3 oz	193	23	0	7	7	2

FOOD	PORTION	CAL	PRO	VIT C	FOL	CA	IR
short loin top loin, lean & fat, trim 0″, Choice; broiled	1 steak (5.4 oz)	353	43	0	12	13	4
short loin top loin, lean & fat, trim 0″, Select; broiled	1 steak (5.4 oz)	309	44	0	12	13	4
short loin top loin, lean & fat, trim ¼″, Choice, raw	1 steak (8.3 oz)	611	44	0	14	14	4
short loin top loin, lean & fat, trim ¼″, Choice; broiled	3 oz	253	22	0	6	8	2
short loin top loin, lean & fat, trim ¼″, Choice; broiled	1 steak (6.3 oz)	536	46	0	13	16	4
short loin top loin, lean & fat, trim ¼″, Select; broiled	1 steak (6.3 oz)	473	46	0	13	16	4
short loin top loin, lean & fat, trim ¼″, Prime; broiled	1 steak (6.3 oz)	582	46	0	13	16	4
short loin top loin, lean only, trim 0″, Choice; broiled	1 steak (5.2 oz)	311	43	0	12	12	4
short loin top loin, lean only, trim ¼″, Choice; broiled	1 steak (5.2 oz)	314	42	0	12	12	4
shortribs, lean & fat, Choice; braised	3 oz	400	18	–	4	10	2
t-bone steak, lean & fat, trim ¼″, Choice; broiled	3 oz	253	21	0	6	7	2
t-bone steak, lean only, trim ¼″, Choice; broiled	3 oz	182	24	0	7	6	3
tenderloin, lean & fat, trim ¼″, Choice; broiled	3 oz	259	21	0	5	7	3
tenderloin, lean & fat, trim ¼″, Choice; roasted	3 oz	288	20	0	7	8	3

FOOD	PORTION	CAL	PRO	VIT C	FOL	CA	IR
tenderloin, lean & fat, trim ¼", Prime; broiled	3 oz	270	21	0	5	7	3
tenderloin, lean & fat, trim ¼", Select; roasted	3 oz	275	21	0	6	8	3
tenderloin, lean & fat, trim ¼", raw	1 oz	80	7	0	2	2	1
tenderloin, lean & fat, trim 0", Choice; broiled	3 oz	208	23	0	6	6	3
tenderloin, lean & fat, trim 0", Select; broiled	3 oz	194	23	0	6	6	3
tenderloin, lean only, trim 0", Select; broiled	3 oz	170	24	0	6	6	3
tenderloin, lean only, trim ¼", Choice; broiled	3 oz	188	24	0	6	6	3
tenderloin, lean only, trim ¼", Select; broiled	3 oz	169	24	0	6	6	3
tip round, lean & fat, trim ¼", Choice; roasted	3 oz	210	23	0	6	5	2
tip round, lean & fat, trim ¼", Prime; roasted	3 oz	233	22	0	6	5	2
tip round, lean & fat, trim ¼", Select; roasted	3 oz	191	23	0	6	5	2
tip round, lean & fat, trim 0", Choice; roasted	3 oz	170	24	0	7	5	2
tip round, lean & fat, trim 0", Select; roasted	3 oz	158	24	0	7	4	2
top round, lean & fat, trim ¼", Choice; braised	3 oz	221	29	0	7	4	3
top round, lean & fat, trim ¼", Choice; broiled	3 oz	190	26	0	10	6	2
top round, lean & fat, trim ¼", Choice; fried	3 oz	235	28	0	10	5	2
top round, lean & fat, trim ¼", Prime; broiled	3 oz	195	26	0	10	5	2

FOOD	PORTION	CAL	PRO	VIT C	FOL	CA	IR
top round, lean & fat, trim ¼", Select; braised	3 oz	199	29	0	7	4	3
top round, lean & fat, trim ¼", Select; broiled	3 oz	175	26	0	10	6	2
top round, lean & fat, trim ¼", raw	1 oz	50	6	0	2	1	1
top round, lean & fat, trim 0", Choice: braised	3 oz	184	30	0	8	3	3
top round, lean & fat, trim 0", Select; braised	3 oz	170	30	0	8	3	3
top sirloin, lean & fat, trim 0", Choice; broiled	3 oz	194	25	0	8	10	3
top sirloin, lean & fat, trim 0", Select; broiled	3 oz	166	25	0	6	9	3
top sirloin, lean & fat, trim ¼", Choice; broiled	3 oz	228	23	0	8	10	3
top sirloin, lean & fat, trim ¼", Choice; fried	3 oz	277	24	0	7	10	3
top sirloin, lean & fat, trim ¼", Select; broiled	3 oz	208	24	0	8	10	3
tripe, raw	4 oz	111	16	4	2	–	2
FROZEN patties, raw	4 oz	319	26	0	8	9	2
patties; broiled medium	3 oz	240	21	0	8	9	2

BEEF DISHES

FOOD	PORTION	CAL	PRO	VIT C	FOL	CA	IR
HOME RECIPE stew w/ vegetables	1 cup	220	16	17	–	29	3
TAKE-OUT roast beef sandwich w/ cheese	1	402	32	0	41	183	5
roast beef sandwich, plain	1	346	22	2	40	54	4
roast beef submarine sandwich w/ tomato, lettuce, mayonnaise	1	411	29	6	45	41	3

FOOD	PORTION	CAL	PRO	VIT C	FOL	CA	IR
steak sandwich w/ tomato, lettuce, salt, mayonnaise	1	459	30	6	89	91	5

BEEFALO

raw	1 oz	41	7	2	4	5	1
roasted	3 oz	160	26	8	15	21	3

BEER AND ALE

beer, light	12 oz. can	100	tr	0	15	18	tr
beer, regular	12 oz. can	146	1	0	21	18	tr

BEETS

CANNED							
harvard	½ cup	89	1	3	–	13	tr
pickled	½ cup	75	1	3	–	13	tr
sliced	½ cup	27	1	–	–	–	2

FRESH							
beet greens, raw; chopped	½ cup	4	tr	6	–	23	1
beet greens, raw	½ cup	4	tr	6	–	23	1
beet greens; cooked	½ cup	20	2	18	–	82	1
cooked	½ cup	26	1	5	45	9	1
raw; sliced	½ cup	30	1	8	63	11	1

JUICE							
beet juice	3½ oz	36	1	3	–	–	–

BISCUIT

biscuit	1 (1 oz)	100	2	tr	–	47	1

MIX							
biscuit	1 (1 oz)	95	2	tr	–	58	1

REFRIGERATED							
biscuit	1 (¾ oz)	65	1	0	–	4	1

FOOD	PORTION	CAL	PRO	VIT C	FOL	CA	IR
TAKE-OUT							
plain	1	276	4	0	6	90	2
w/ egg	1	315	11	0	29	154	3
w/ egg & bacon	1	457	17	3	29	189	4
w/ egg & sausage	1	582	19	tr	40	155	4
w/ egg & steak	1	474	18	tr	28	138	5
w/ egg, cheese & bacon	1	477	16	2	37	164	3
w/ ham	1	387	13	tr	8	161	3
w/ sausage	1	485	12	tr	9	128	3
w/ steak	1	456	13	tr	11	115	4
BISON							
raw	1 oz	31	6	–	–	2	1
roasted	3 oz	122	24	–	–	7	3
BLACK BEANS							
DRIED							
cooked	1 cup	227	15	0	256	47	4
raw	1 cup	661	42	0	862	239	10
BLACKBERRIES							
CANNED							
in heavy syrup	½ cup	118	2	4	34	27	1
FRESH							
blackberries	½ cup	37	1	15	–	23	tr
FROZEN							
unsweetened	1 cup	97	2	5	51	44	1
BLUEBERRIES							
CANNED							
in heavy syrup	1 cup	225	2	3	4	7	1
FRESH							
blueberries	1 cup	82	1	19	9	9	tr

FOOD	PORTION	CAL	PRO	VIT C	FOL	CA	IR
FROZEN							
unsweetened	1 cup	78	1	4	10	12	tr
BLUEFISH							
FRESH							
raw	3 oz	105	17	–	2	6	tr
BOAR							
wild, raw	1 oz	35	6	–	–	3	–
wild; roasted	3 oz	136	24	–	–	13	–
BORAGE							
FRESH							
cooked; chopped	3½ oz	25	2	33	–	102	4
raw; chopped	½ cup	9	1	15	–	41	1
BOYSENBERRIES							
CANNED							
in heavy syrup	1 cup	226	3	16	88	23	1
FROZEN							
unsweetened	1 cup	66	1	4	84	36	1
BRAINS							
beef; pan-fried	3 oz	167	11	3	5	8	2
beef; simmered	3 oz	136	9	1	6	8	2
lamb; braised	3 oz	124	11	10	4	10	1
lamb; fried	3 oz	232	14	20	6	18	2
pork, raw	3 oz	108	–	–	–	9	–
pork; braised	3 oz	117	10	12	–	8	2
veal; braised	3 oz	115	10	11	3	13	1
veal; fried	3 oz	181	12	12	5	9	1
BRAN							
corn; cooked	⅓ cup	56	2	0	1	11	tr

FOOD	PORTION	CAL	PRO	VIT C	FOL	CA	IR
oat, dry	½ cup	116	8	0	24	27	3
oat; cooked	½ cup	44	4	0	7	11	tr
rice, dry	⅓ cup	88	4	0	18	16	5
wheat, dry	½ cup	65	5	0	24	22	3

BRAZIL NUTS

FOOD	PORTION	CAL	PRO	VIT C	FOL	CA	IR
dried, unblanched	1 oz	186	4	tr	1	50	1

BREAD

FOOD	PORTION	CAL	PRO	VIT C	FOL	CA	IR
CANNED							
boston brown	1 slice	95	2	0	–	41	1
HOME RECIPE							
hush puppies	5 (2.7 oz)	256	5	0	21	69	1
READY-TO-EAT							
cracked wheat	1 slice	65	2	tr	–	16	1
cracked wheat; toasted	1 slice	65	2	tr	–	16	1
french	1 loaf (1 lb)	454	43	tr	–	499	14
french	1 slice (1.2 oz)	100	3	tr	–	39	1
italian	1 slice (1 oz)	85	3	0	–	5	1
italian	1 loaf (1 lb)	454	41	0	–	77	13
oatmeal	1 slice	65	2	0	–	15	1
pita	1 (2 oz)	165	6	0	–	49	1
pumpernickel	1 slice	80	3	0	–	23	1
raisin	1 slice	65	2	tr	–	25	1
rye	1 slice	65	2	0	–	20	1
vienna	1 slice (.9 oz)	70	3	tr	–	28	1
wheat	1 slice	65	2	tr	–	32	1
white	1 slice	65	2	tr	–	32	1

FOOD	PORTION	CAL	PRO	VIT C	FOL	CA	IR
white; cubed	1 cup	80	2	tr	–	38	1
whole wheat	1 slice	70	3	tr	–	20	1

BREAD CRUMBS

dry	1 cup	390	13	0	–	122	4
fresh	1 cup	120	4	tr	–	57	1

BREADFRUIT

fresh	¼ small	99	1	28	–	17	1
seeds, raw	1 oz	54	2	2	–	10	1
seeds, roasted	1 oz	59	2	–	–	24	tr
seeds; cooked	1 oz	48	2	–	–	12	tr

BREADNUTTREE SEEDS

dried	1 oz	104	2	–	13	27	1

BREAKFAST DRINKS

orange drink powder; as prep w/ water	6 oz	86	0	91	107	46	tr
orange drink, powder	3 rounded tsp	93	0	98	116	46	tr

BROAD BEANS

CANNED broad beans	1 cup	183	14	5	84	67	3
DRIED cooked	1 cup	186	13	1	177	62	3
raw	1 cup	511	39	2	634	154	10
FRESH cooked	3½ oz	56	5	20	–	18	2

BROCCOLI

FRESH chopped, cooked	½ cup	23	2	49	39	89	1

FOOD	PORTION	CAL	PRO	VIT C	FOL	CA	IR
raw; chopped	½ cup	12	1	41	31	21	tr
FROZEN							
chopped, cooked	½ cup	25	3	37	52	47	1
spears; cooked	10 oz pkg	69	8	100	76	127	2
spears; cooked	½ cup	25	3	37	28	127	1

BROWNIE

FOOD	PORTION	CAL	PRO	VIT C	FOL	CA	IR
HOME RECIPE							
w/ nuts	1 (.8 oz)	95	1	tr	–	9	tr
READY-TO-EAT							
w/ nuts	1 (1 oz)	100	1	tr	–	13	1
w/o nuts	1 (2 oz)	243	3	3	4	25	1

BRUSSELS SPROUTS

FOOD	PORTION	CAL	PRO	VIT C	FOL	CA	IR
FRESH							
cooked	½ cup	30	2	48	47	28	1
cooked	1 sprout	8	1	13	13	7	tr
raw	½ cup	19	1	37	27	18	1
raw	1 sprout	8	1	16	12	8	tr
FROZEN							
cooked	½ cup	33	3	36	79	19	1

BUCKWHEAT

FOOD	PORTION	CAL	PRO	VIT C	FOL	CA	IR
flour, whole groat	1 cup	402	15	0	64	–	–
groats, roasted: uncooked	½ cup	283	10	0	35	14	2
groats, roasted; cooked	½ cup	91	3	0	14	7	tr

BUFFALO

FOOD	PORTION	CAL	PRO	VIT C	FOL	CA	IR
water, raw	1 oz	28	6	–	2	3	tr
water; roasted	3 oz	111	23	–	8	13	2

FOOD	PORTION	CAL	PRO	VIT C	FOL	CA	IR
BULGUR							
cooked	½ cup	76	3	0	17	9	tr
uncooked	½ cup	239	9	0	19	25	2
BURBOT (FISH)							
FRESH							
raw	3 oz	76	16	–	–	43	1
BURDOCK ROOT							
cooked	1 cup	110	3	–	–	62	1
raw	1 cup	85	2	4	–	48	1
BUTTER							
REGULAR							
butter	1 pat	36	tr	0	tr	1	tr
butter	1 stick (4 oz)	813	1	0	3	27	tr
butter oil	1 cup	1795	1	–	–	–	–
butter oil	1 tbsp	112	tr	–	–	–	–
clarified butter	3½ oz	876	tr	0	–	tr	–
WHIPPED							
butter	1 pat	27	tr	–	tr	1	tr
butter	4 oz	542	1	0	2	18	tr
BUTTERBUR							
CANNED							
fuki, chopped	1 cup	3	tr	15	–	42	1
FRESH							
raw fuki	1 cup	13	tr	30	–	97	tr
BUTTERFISH							
raw	3 oz	124	–	–	–	tr	–
BUTTERNUTS							
dried	1 oz	174	7	–	–	15	1

FOOD	PORTION	CAL	PRO	VIT C	FOL	CA	IR
CABBAGE							
FRESH							
chinese, pak-choi, raw; shredded	½ cup	5	1	16	–	37	tr
chinese, pak-choi; shredded, cooked	½ cup	10	1	22	–	79	1
chinese, pe-tsai, raw; shredded	1 cup	12	1	21	60	58	tr
chinese, pe-tsai; shredded, cooked	1 cup	16	2	19	64	38	tr
green, raw; shredded	½ cup	8	tr	17	20	16	tr
green, raw; shredded	1 head (2 lbs)	215	11	429	515	424	5
green; shredded, cooked	½ cup	16	1	18	15	25	tr
red, raw; shredded	½ cup	10	tr	20	7	18	tr
red; shredded, cooked	½ cup	16	1	26	9	28	tr
savoy, raw; shredded	½ cup	10	1	11	–	12	tr
savoy; shredded, cooked	½ cup	18	1	12	–	22	tr
HOME RECIPE							
coleslaw	½ cup	42	1	20	16	27	tr
coleslaw w/ dressing	¾ cup	147	1	8	39	34	tr
CAKE							
carrot w/ cream cheese icing	1 cake 10″ diam	6175	63	23	–	707	21
carrot w/ cream cheese icing	1/16 of cake	385	4	1	–	44	1
fruitcake, dark	1 cake 7½″ × 2¼″	5185	74	504	–	1293	38
fruitcake, dark	⅔ slice	165	2	16	–	41	1
pound	1 loaf 8½″ × 3½″	1935	33	1	–	146	9

FOOD	PORTION	CAL	PRO	VIT C	FOL	CA	IR
pound cake	1 slice (1 oz)	120	2	tr	–	20	1
sheet cake w/ white frosting	⅑ of cake	445	4	tr	–	61	1
sheet cake w/ white frosting	1 cake 9" sq	4020	37	2	–	548	11
sheet cake w/o frosting	1 cake 9" sq	2830	35	2	–	497	12
sheet cake w/o frosting	⅑ of cake	315	4	tr	–	55	1
MIX angelfood	1 cake 9¾" diam	1510	38	0	–	527	3
angelfood	1/12 of cake	125	3	0	–	44	tr
crumb coffeecake	1 cake 7¾" × 5⅝"	1385	27	1	–	262	7
crumb coffeecake	⅙ of cake	230	5	tr	–	44	1
devil's food cupcake w/ chocolate frosting	1	120	2	tr	–	21	1
devil's food w/ chocolate frosting	1 cake 9" diam	3755	49	1	–	653	22
devil's food w/ chocolate frosting	1/16 of cake	235	3	tr	–	41	1
gingerbread	1 cake 8" sq	1575	18	1	–	513	11
gingerbread	⅑ cake	175	2	tr	–	57	1
yellow w/ chocolate frosting; as prep	1 cake 9" diam	3735	45	1	–	1008	16
yellow w/ chocolate frosting; as prep	1/16 of cake	235	3	tr	–	63	1
READY-TO-USE cheesecake	1 cake 9" diam	3350	60	56	–	622	5
cheesecake	1/12 of cake	280	5	5	–	52	tr

FOOD	PORTION	CAL	PRO	VIT C	FOL	CA	IR
pound cake	1 cake (8½" × 3½" × 3")	1935	26	0	–	146	8
pound cake	1 slice (1 oz)	110	2	0	–	8	1
white w/ white frosting	1 cake 9" diam	4170	43	0	–	536	16
white w/ white frosting	1/16 cake	260	3	0	–	33	1
yellow w/ chocolate frosting	1 cake 9" diam	3895	40	0	–	366	20
yellow w/ chocolate frosting	1/16 cake	245	2	0	–	23	1
SNACK devil's food w/ creme filling	1 (1 oz)	105	1	0	–	21	1
sponge w/ creme filling	1 (1.5 oz)	155	1	0	–	14	1
toaster pastries	1 (1.9 oz)	210	2	4	–	104	2

CANADIAN BACON

FOOD	PORTION	CAL	PRO	VIT C	FOL	CA	IR
unheated	2 slices (1.9 oz)	89	12	12	2	5	tr

CANDY

FOOD	PORTION	CAL	PRO	VIT C	FOL	CA	IR
candy corn	1 oz	105	tr	0	–	2	tr
caramels, chocolate	1 oz	115	1	tr	–	42	tr
caramels, plain	1 oz	115	1	tr	–	42	tr
chocolate	1 oz	145	2	tr	–	50	tr
chocolate crisp	1 oz	140	2	tr	–	48	tr
chocolate w/ almonds	1 oz	150	3	tr	–	65	1
chocolate w/ peanuts	1 oz	155	4	tr	–	49	tr
dark chocolate	1 oz	150	1	tr	–	7	1
fudge, chocolate	1 oz	115	1	tr	–	22	tr
fudge, vanilla	1 oz	115	1	tr	–	22	tr

FOOD	PORTION	CAL	PRO	VIT C	FOL	CA	IR
gum drops	1 oz	100	tr	0	–	2	tr
hard candy	1 oz	110	0	0	–	tr	tr
jelly beans	1 oz	105	tr	0	–	1	tr
marshmallow	1 oz	90	1	0	–	1	1
marzipan	3½ oz	497	8	2	–	43	2
mint fondant	1 oz	105	tr	0	–	2	tr
nougat nut cream	3½ oz	342	4	–	–	13	4

CANTALOUP

FOOD	PORTION	CAL	PRO	VIT C	FOL	CA	IR
cubed	1 cup	57	1	68	27	17	tr
fresh	½	94	2	113	46	28	1

CARAMBOLA

FOOD	PORTION	CAL	PRO	VIT C	FOL	CA	IR
fresh	1	42	1	27	–	6	tr

CARAWAY

FOOD	PORTION	CAL	PRO	VIT C	FOL	CA	IR
seed	1 tsp	7	tr	–	–	14	tr

CARDAMON

FOOD	PORTION	CAL	PRO	VIT C	FOL	CA	IR
ground	1 tsp	6	tr	–	–	8	tr

CARDOON

FOOD	PORTION	CAL	PRO	VIT C	FOL	CA	IR
FRESH							
cardoon; cooked	3½ oz	22	1	2	–	72	1
raw; shredded	½ cup	36	1	2	–	62	1

CARIBOU

FOOD	PORTION	CAL	PRO	VIT C	FOL	CA	IR
raw	1 oz	36	6	1	1	5	1
roasted	3 oz	142	25	3	4	19	5

CARISSA

FOOD	PORTION	CAL	PRO	VIT C	FOL	CA	IR
fresh	1	12	tr	8	–	2	tr

FOOD	PORTION	CAL	PRO	VIT C	FOL	CA	IR
CAROB							
carob mix	3 tsp	45	tr	0	–	–	1
carob mix; as prep w/ whole milk	9 oz	195	8	2	12	291	1
flour	1 cup	185	5	tr	30	359	3
flour	1 tbsp	14	tr	0	2	28	tr
CARP							
FRESH							
cooked	3 oz	138	19	1	–	44	1
cooked	1 fillet (6 oz)	276	39	3	–	89	3
raw	3 oz	108	15	1	–	15	1
CARROTS							
CANNED							
slices	½ cup	17	tr	2	7	19	tr
FRESH							
raw	1 (2.5 oz)	31	1	7	10	19	tr
raw; shredded	½ cup	24	1	5	8	15	tr
slices; cooked	½ cup	35	1	2	11	24	tr
FROZEN							
slices; cooked	½ cup	26	1	2	8	21	tr
JUICE							
canned	6 oz	73	2	16	7	44	1
CASABA							
cubed	1 cup	45	2	27	–	9	1
fresh	⅒	43	1	26	–	8	1
CASHEWS							
cashew butter w/o salt	1 tbsp	94	3	0	11	7	1
dry roasted	1 oz	163	4	0	20	13	2

FOOD	PORTION	CAL	PRO	VIT C	FOL	CA	IR
dry roasted, salted	1 oz	163	4	0	20	13	2
oil roasted	1 oz	163	5	0	19	12	1
oil roasted, salted	1 oz	163	5	0	19	12	1

CASSAVA

FRESH
| raw | 3½ oz | 120 | 3 | 48 | – | 91 | 4 |

CATFISH

| channel, raw | 3 oz | 99 | 15 | – | – | 34 | 1 |
| channel; breaded & fried | 3 oz | 194 | 15 | 0 | – | 37 | 1 |

CATSUP

| catsup | 1 tbsp | 16 | tr | 2 | 2 | 3 | tr |

CAULIFLOWER

FRESH
| cooked | ½ cup | 15 | 1 | 34 | 32 | 17 | tr |
| raw | ½ cup | 12 | 1 | 36 | 33 | 14 | tr |

FROZEN
| cooked | ½ cup | 17 | 1 | 28 | 37 | 15 | tr |

CAVIAR

black granular	1 tbsp	40	4	–	–	–	–
black granular	1 oz	71	7	–	–	–	–
red granular	1 tbsp	40	4	–	–	–	–
red granular	1 oz	71	7	–	–	–	–

CELERIAC

FRESH
| cooked | 3½ oz | 25 | 1 | 4 | – | 26 | tr |
| raw | ½ cup | 31 | 1 | 6 | – | 34 | 1 |

FOOD	PORTION	CAL	PRO	VIT C	FOL	CA	IR
CELERY							
DRIED							
seed	1 tsp	8	tr	–	–	35	1
FRESH							
diced, cooked	½ cup	11	tr	4	16	27	tr
raw	1 stalk (2 oz)	6	tr	3	11	14	tr
raw; diced	½ cup	9	tr	4	17	22	tr
CELTUCE							
raw	3½ oz	22	1	20	–	39	1
CEREAL							
COOKED							
corn grits, instant; as prep	1 pkg (.8 oz)	82	–	–	1	7	–
farina, dry	1 tbsp	40	1	–	3	2	tr
farina; cooked	¾ cup	87	3	–	4	3	tr
oatmeal, instant; cooked w/o salt	1 cup	145	6	0	–	19	2
oatmeal, quick; cooked w/o salt	1 cup	145	6	0	–	19	2
oatmeal, regular; cooked w/o salt	1 cup	145	6	0	–	19	2
oatmeal, dry	1 cup	311	13	–	26	42	3
oatmeal; cooked	1 cup	145	6	–	9	20	2
READY-TO-EAT							
all bran	⅓ cup (1 oz)	70	4	15	–	23	5
bran flakes	¾ cup (1 oz)	90	4	0	–	14	8
corn flakes	1¼ cup (1 oz)	110	2	15	–	1	2
shredded wheat	1 biscuit	83	3	–	12	10	1

FOOD	PORTION	CAL	PRO	VIT C	FOL	CA	IR
sugar-coated corn flakes	¾ cup (1 oz)	110	1	15	–	1	2

CHAYOTE

FRESH

cooked	1 cup	38	1	13	–	21	tr
raw	1 (7 oz)	49	2	22	–	39	1
raw; cut up	1 cup	32	1	15	–	25	1

CHEESE

NATURAL

bel paese	3½ oz	391	25	–	–	604	–
blue	1 oz	100	6	0	10	150	tr
blue; crumbled	1 cup	477	29	0	49	712	tr
brick	1 oz	105	7	0	6	191	tr
brie	1 oz	95	8	0	18	52	tr
camembert	1 oz	85	6	0	18	110	tr
camembert	1 wedge (1⅓ oz)	114	8	0	24	147	tr
caraway	1 oz	107	7	0	–	191	–
cheddar	1 oz	114	7	0	5	204	tr
cheddar; shredded	1 cup	455	28	0	21	815	1
cheshire	1 oz	110	7	0	–	182	tr
colby	1 oz	112	7	0	–	194	tr
edam	1 oz	101	7	0	5	207	tr
emmentaler	3½ oz	403	29	1	tr	1020	tr
feta	1 oz	75	4	0	–	140	tr
fontina	1 oz	110	7	0	–	156	tr
gjetost	1 oz	132	3	0	1	113	–
gorgonzola	3½ oz	376	19	–	tr	612	tr
gouda	1 oz	101	7	0	6	198	tr

FOOD	PORTION	CAL	PRO	VIT C	FOL	CA	IR
gruyere	1 oz	117	8	0	3	287	–
limburger	1 oz	93	8	0	16	141	tr
monterey	1 oz	106	7	0	–	212	tr
mozzarella	1 oz	80	6	0	1	147	tr
mozzarella	1 lb	1276	88	0	32	2345	1
mozzarella, low moisture	1 oz	90	6	0	2	163	tr
mozzarella, part skim	1 oz	72	7	0	2	183	tr
mozzarella, part skim, low moisture	1 oz	79	8	0	3	207	tr
muenster	1 oz	104	7	0	3	203	tr
parmesan, hard	1 oz	111	10	0	2	336	tr
parmesan; grated	1 tbsp	23	2	0	tr	69	tr
parmesan; grated	1 oz	129	12	0	2	390	tr
port du salut	1 oz	100	7	0	5	184	–
provolone	1 oz	100	7	0	3	214	tr
quark, 20% fat	3½ oz	116	13	1	tr	85	tr
quark, 40% fat	3½ oz	167	11	1	–	95	tr
quark, made w/ skim milk	3½ oz	78	14	1	tr	92	tr
ricotta	½ cup	216	14	0	–	257	tr
ricotta	1 cup	428	28	0	–	509	1
ricotta, part skim	½ cup	171	14	0	–	337	1
ricotta, part skim	1 cup	340	28	0	–	669	1
romadur, 40% fat	3½ oz	289	23	–	–	403	–
romano	1 oz	110	9	0	2	302	–
roquefort	1 oz	105	6	0	14	188	tr
swiss	1 oz	107	8	0	2	272	tr
tilsit	1 oz	96	7	0	–	198	tr
PROCESSED american	1 oz	106	6	0	2	174	tr

FOOD	PORTION	CAL	PRO	VIT C	FOL	CA	IR
american, cheese food	1 oz	93	6	0	–	163	tr
american, cheese food	1 pkg (8 oz)	745	45	0	–	1303	2
american, cheese food, cold pack	1 oz	94	6	0	2	141	tr
american, cheese food, cold pack	1 pkg (8 oz)	752	45	0	12	1129	2
american, cheese spread	1 oz	82	5	0	2	159	tr
american, cheese spread	1 jar (5 oz)	412	23	0	10	798	tr
pimento	1 oz	106	6	–	2	174	tr
swiss	1 oz	95	7	0	–	219	tr
swiss, cheese food	1 oz	92	6	0	–	205	tr
swiss, cheese food	1 pkg (8 oz)	734	50	0	–	1642	1

CHERIMOYA

FOOD	PORTION	CAL	PRO	VIT C	FOL	CA	IR
fresh	1	515	7	49	–	126	3

CHERRIES

CANNED

FOOD	PORTION	CAL	PRO	VIT C	FOL	CA	IR
sour in heavy syrup	½ cup	232	2	5	19	26	3
sour in light syrup	½ cup	189	2	5	19	26	3
sour water packed	1 cup	87	2	5	20	26	3
sweet in heavy syrup	½ cup	107	1	5	–	12	tr
sweet in light syrup	½ cup	85	1	5	–	12	tr
sweet juice pack	½ cup	68	1	3	–	17	1
sweet water pack	½ cup	57	1	3	–	13	tr

FRESH

FOOD	PORTION	CAL	PRO	VIT C	FOL	CA	IR
sour	1 cup	51	1	10	8	16	tr
sweet	10	49	1	5	3	10	tr

FOOD	PORTION	CAL	PRO	VIT C	FOL	CA	IR
FROZEN							
sour unsweetened	1 cup	72	1	3	7	20	1
sweet sweetened	1 cup	232	3	3	–	31	1
CHERVIL							
seed	1 tsp	1	tr	–	–	8	tr
CHESTNUTS							
chinese dried	1 oz	103	2	–	–	8	1
chinese, raw	1 oz	64	1	10	–	5	tr
chinese; cooked	1 oz	44	1	–	–	3	tr
chinese; roasted	1 oz	68	1	–	–	5	tr
cooked	1 oz	37	1	–	–	13	tr
dried; peeled	1 oz	105	1	–	–	18	1
japanese, dried	1 oz	102	1	17	–	20	1
japanese, raw	1 oz	44	1	8	–	9	tr
japanese; roasted	1 oz	57	1	8	–	10	1
japanese; cooked	1 oz	16	tr	–	–	3	tr
raw; peeled	1 oz	56	tr	–	–	5	tr
roasted	1 oz	70	1	7	10	8	tr
roasted	1 cup	350	5	37	100	42	1
CHIA SEEDS							
dried	1 oz	134	5	–	–	150	3
CHICKEN							
CANNED							
chicken spread	1 tbsp	25	2	–	–	16	tr
chicken spread	1 oz	55	4	–	–	35	1
chicken spread, barbeque flavored	1 oz	55	4	1	–	35	1
w/ broth	1 can (5 oz)	234	31	3	–	20	2

FOOD	PORTION	CAL	PRO	VIT C	FOL	CA	IR
w/ broth	½ can (2.5 oz)	117	15	1	–	10	1
FRESH							
broiler/fryer breast w/ skin; batter dipped, fried	½ breast (4.9 oz)	364	35	0	8	28	1
broiler/fryer thigh w/ skin; roasted	1 (2.2 oz)	153	16	0	4	8	1
broiler/fryer back meat w/o skin, raw	1 oz	42	6	1	3	5	tr
broiler/fryer back w/ skin, raw	½ back (3.5 oz)	316	14	2	6	13	1
broiler/fryer back w/ skin; batter dipped, fried	½ back (2.5 oz)	238	16	0	6	17	1
broiler/fryer back w/ skin; floured, fried	1.5 oz	146	12	0	3	10	1
broiler/fryer back w/ skin; roasted	1 oz	96	8	0	2	7	tr
broiler/fryer back w/ skin; stewed	½ back (2.1 oz)	158	14	0	3	11	1
broiler/fryer back w/o skin; fried	½ back (2 oz)	167	17	0	5	15	1
broiler/fryer breast w/ skin, raw	3.1 oz	150	18	1	4	9	1
broiler/fryer breast w/ skin; batter dipped, fried	2.9 oz	218	21	0	5	17	1
broiler/fryer breast w/ skin; roasted	½ breast (3.4 oz)	193	29	0	3	14	1
broiler/fryer breast w/ skin; roasted	2 oz	115	17	0	2	8	1
broiler/fryer breast w/ skin; stewed	½ breast (3.9 oz)	202	30	0	3	14	1
broiler/fryer breast w/o skin, raw	½ breast (4 oz)	129	27	2	5	13	1
broiler/fryer breast w/o skin; fried	½ breast (3 oz)	161	29	0	4	14	1

FOOD	PORTION	CAL	PRO	VIT C	FOL	CA	IR
broiler/fryer breast w/o skin; roasted	½ breast (3 oz)	142	27	0	3	13	1
broiler/fryer breast w/o skin; stewed	2 oz	86	17	0	2	7	1
broiler/fryer breast w/ skin, raw	½ breast (5.1 oz)	250	30	2	6	16	1
broiler/fryer dark meat w/ skin, raw	½ chicken (9.3 oz)	630	49	6	19	29	3
broiler/fryer dark meat w/ skin; batter dipped, fried	5.9 oz	497	36	0	15	36	2
broiler/fryer dark meat w/ skin; floured, fried	3.9 oz	313	30	0	9	19	2
broiler/fryer dark meat w/ skin; roasted	3.5 oz	256	26	0	7	15	1
broiler/fryer dark meat w/ skin; stewed	3.9 oz	256	26	0	7	15	1
broiler/fryer dark meat w/o skin, raw	3.8 oz	136	22	3	11	13	1
broiler/fryer dark meat w/o skin; fried	1 cup (5 oz)	334	41	0	12	25	2
broiler/fryer dark meat w/o skin; roasted	1 cup (5 oz)	286	38	0	11	21	2
broiler/fryer dark meat w/o skin; stewed	1 cup (5 oz)	269	36	0	10	20	2
broiler/fryer dark meat w/o skin; stewed	3 oz	165	22	0	6	12	1
broiler/fryer drumstick w/ skin, raw	1 (2.6 oz)	117	14	2	6	8	1
broiler/fryer drumstick w/ skin; batter dipped, fried	1 (2.6 oz)	193	16	0	6	12	1
broiler/fryer drumstick w/ skin; floured, fried	1 (1.7 oz)	120	13	0	4	6	1
broiler/fryer drumstick w/ skin; roasted	1 (1.8 oz)	112	14	0	4	6	1

FOOD	PORTION	CAL	PRO	VIT C	FOL	CA	IR
broiler/fryer drumstick w/ skin; stewed	1 (2 oz)	116	14	0	4	7	1
broiler/fryer drumstick w/o skin, raw	1 (2.2 oz)	74	13	2	6	7	1
broiler/fryer drumstick w/o skin; fried	1 (1.5 oz)	82	12	0	4	5	1
broiler/fryer drumstick w/o skin; roasted	1 (1.5 oz)	76	12	0	4	5	1
broiler/fryer drumstick w/o skin; stewed	1 (1.6 oz)	78	13	0	4	5	1
broiler/fryer leg w/ skin, raw	1 (5.6 oz)	312	30	4	19	17	2
broiler/fryer leg w/ skin; batter dipped, fried	1 (5.5 oz)	431	34	0	14	28	2
broiler/fryer leg w/ skin; roasted	1 (4 oz)	265	30	0	8	14	2
broiler/fryer leg w/ skin; stewed	1 (4.4 oz)	275	30	0	8	14	2
broiler/fryer leg w/o skin, raw	1 (4.6 oz)	156	26	4	13	14	1
broiler/fryer leg w/o skin; fried	1 (3.3 oz)	195	27	0	8	12	1
broiler/fryer leg w/o skin; roasted	1 (3.3 oz)	182	26	0	8	12	1
broiler/fryer leg w/o skin; stewed	1 (3.5 oz)	187	26	0	8	11	1
broiler/fryer leg w/ skin; floured, fried	1 (3.9 oz)	285	30	0	9	15	2
broiler/fryer light meat w/ skin, raw	½ chicken (6.8 oz)	362	39	2	8	22	2
broiler/fryer light meat w/ skin, raw	4.1 oz	216	24	1	5	13	1
broiler/fryer light meat w/ skin; batter dipped, fried	4 oz	312	27	0	7	22	1

FOOD	PORTION	CAL	PRO	VIT C	FOL	CA	IR
broiler/fryer light meat w/ skin; floured, fried	2.7 oz	192	24	0	3	12	1
broiler/fryer light meat w/ skin; roasted	2.8 oz	175	23	0	3	12	1
broiler/fryer light meat w/ skin; stewed	3.2 oz	181	9	0	3	11	1
broiler/fryer light meat w/o skin, raw	3.1 oz	100	20	1	4	10	1
broiler/fryer light meat w/o skin; fried	1 cup (5 oz)	268	46	0	6	22	2
broiler/fryer light meat w/o skin; roasted	1 cup (5 oz)	242	43	0	5	21	1
broiler/fryer light meat w/o skin; stewed	1 cup (5 oz)	223	40	0	5	18	1
broiler/fryer neck w/ skin, raw	1 (1.8 oz)	148	7	1	2	9	1
broiler/fryer neck w/ skin; stewed	1 (1.3 oz)	94	7	0	1	10	1
broiler/fryer neck w/o skin, raw	1 (.7 oz)	31	4	1	2	5	tr
broiler/fryer neck w/o skin; stewed	1 (.6 oz)	32	4	0	tr	8	tr
broiler/fryer skin, raw	from ½ chicken (2.8 oz)	275	11	0	2	8	1
broiler/fryer skin; batter dipped, fried	from ½ chicken (6.7 oz)	748	20	0	17	49	3
broiler/fryer skin; batter dipped, fried	4 oz	449	12	0	10	29	2
broiler/fryer skin; floured, fried	1 oz	166	6	0	1	5	1
broiler/fryer skin; floured, fried	from ½ chicken (2 oz)	281	24	0	2	8	1

FOOD	PORTION	CAL	PRO	VIT C	FOL	CA	IR
broiler/fryer skin; roasted	from ½ chicken (2 oz)	254	11	0	1	8	1
broiler/fryer skin; stewed	from ½ chicken (2.5 oz)	261	11	0	1	9	1
broiler/fryer thigh w/ skin; floured, fried	1 (2.2 oz)	162	17	0	5	8	1
broiler/fryer thigh w/ skin, raw	1 (3.3 oz)	199	16	2	7	9	1
broiler/fryer thigh w/ skin; batter dipped, fried	1 (3 oz)	238	19	0	8	16	1
broiler/fryer thigh w/ skin; stewed	1 (2.4 oz)	158	16	0	4	8	1
broiler/fryer thigh w/o skin, raw	1 (2.4 oz)	82	14	2	7	7	1
broiler/fryer thigh w/o skin; fried	1 (1.8 oz)	113	15	0	4	7	1
broiler/fryer thigh w/o skin; roasted	1 (1.8 oz)	109	13	0	4	6	1
broiler/fryer thigh w/o skin; stewed	1 (1.9 oz)	107	14	0	4	6	1
broiler/fryer w/ skin; floured, fried	½ breast (3.4 oz)	218	31	0	4	16	1
broiler/fryer w/o skin, raw	½ chicken (11.5 oz)	392	70	8	24	40	3
broiler/fryer w/o skin; roasted	1 cup (5 oz)	266	41	0	8	21	2
broiler/fryer w/o skin; fried	1 cup	307	43	0	10	24	2
broiler/fryer w/o skin; stewed	1 cup (5 oz)	248	38	0	8	19	2
broiler/fryer w/o skin; stewed	1 oz	54	7	0	2	6	tr

FOOD	PORTION	CAL	PRO	VIT C	FOL	CA	IR
broiler/fryer wing w/ skin, raw	1 (1.7 oz)	109	9	tr	2	6	tr
broiler/fryer wing w/ skin; batter dipped, fried	1 (1.7 oz)	159	10	0	3	10	1
broiler/fryer wing w/ skin; floured, fried	1 (1.1 oz)	103	8	0	1	5	tr
broiler/fryer wing w/ skin; roasted	1 (1.2 oz)	99	9	0	1	5	tr
broiler/fryer wing w/ skin; stewed	1 (1.4 oz)	100	9	0	1	5	tr
broiler/fryer w/ skin, neck & giblets, raw	1 chicken (2.3 lbs)	2223	192	28	315	119	14
broiler/fryer w/ skin, neck & giblets; batter dipped, fried	1 chicken (2.3 lbs)	2987	235	4	241	218	18
broiler/fryer w/ skin, neck & giblets; roasted	1 chicken (1.5 lbs)	1598	183	4	201	105	11
broiler/fryer w/ skin, neck & giblets; stewed	1 chicken (1.6 lbs)	1625	184	4	200	104	12
broiler/fryer w/ skin, raw	½ chicken (16.1 oz)	990	86	8	27	51	4
broiler/fryer w/ skin; floured, fried	½ chicken (11 oz)	844	90	0	20	52	4
broiler/fryer w/ skin; fried	½ chicken (16.4 oz)	1347	81	0	35	97	6
broiler/fryer w/ skin; roasted	½ chicken (10.5 oz)	715	82	0	16	45	4
broiler/fryer w/ skin; stewed	½ chicken (11.7 oz)	730	82	0	16	44	4
capon w/ skin, neck & giblets, raw	1 chicken (4.7 lbs)	4987	398	56	575	234	30
capon w/ skin, neck & giblets; roasted	1 chicken (3.1 lbs)	3211	402	6	367	211	25
roaster dark meat w/o skin; roasted	1 cup (5 oz)	250	33	0	9	15	2

FOOD	PORTION	CAL	PRO	VIT C	FOL	CA	IR
roaster light meat w/o skin; roasted	1 cup (5 oz)	214	38	0	5	18	2
roaster w/ skin, neck & giblets, raw	1 chicken (3.3 lbs)	3210	258	36	389	151	21
roaster w/ skin, neck & giblets; roasted	1 chicken (2.4 lbs)	2363	257	4	251	136	17
roaster w/o skin; roasted	1 cup (5 oz)	469	9	0	7	25	2
roaster w/ skin; roasted	½ chicken (1.1 lbs)	1071	115	0	22	58	6
stewing dark meat w/o skin; stewed	1 cup (5 oz)	361	39	0	12	17	2
stewing w/ skin, neck & giblets, raw	1 chicken (2 lbs)	2275	158	28	331	93	14
stewing w/ skin, neck & giblets; stewed	1 chicken (1.3 lbs)	1636	157	3	211	78	11
stewing w/ skin; stewed	½ chicken (9.2 oz)	744	70	0	13	33	4
stewing w/ skin; stewed	6.2 oz	507	34	0	9	22	2
READY-TO-USE chicken roll, light meat	2 oz	90	11	–	–	24	1
chicken roll, light meat	1 pkg (6 oz)	271	33	–	–	73	2
poultry salad sandwich spread	1 tbsp	109	2	0	1	1	tr
poultry salad sandwich spread	1 oz	238	3	0	1	3	tr
TAKE-OUT boneless, w/ barbecue sauce; breaded & fried	6 pieces (4.6 oz)	330	17	tr	28	21	1
boneless, w/ honey; breaded & fried	6 pieces (4 oz)	339	17	tr	11	17	1
boneless, w/ mustard sauce; breaded & fried	6 pieces (4.6 oz)	323	17	tr	12	25	1

FOOD	PORTION	CAL	PRO	VIT C	FOL	CA	IR
boneless, w/ sweet & sour sauce; breaded & fried	6 pieces (4.6 oz)	346	17	tr	12	20	1
breast & wing; breaded & fried	2 pieces (5.7 oz)	494	36	0	9	60	1
drumstick; breaded & fried	2 pieces (5.2 oz)	430	30	0	10	36	2
fillet sandwich w/ cheese, mayonnaise, tomato, lettuce	1	632	29	3	46	258	4
fillet sandwich, plain	1	515	24	9	28	60	5
thigh; breaded & fried	2 pieces (5.2 oz)	430	30	0	10	36	2

CHICKEN DISHES

HOME RECIPE

FOOD	PORTION	CAL	PRO	VIT C	FOL	CA	IR
chicken & noodles	1 cup	365	22	tr	–	26	2
chicken a la king	1 cup	470	27	12	–	127	3

CHICKPEAS

CANNED

FOOD	PORTION	CAL	PRO	VIT C	FOL	CA	IR
chickpeas	1 cup	285	12	9	160	78	3

DRIED

FOOD	PORTION	CAL	PRO	VIT C	FOL	CA	IR
cooked	1 cup	269	15	2	0	80	5
raw	1 cup	729	39	8	1113	211	12

CHICORY

FRESH

FOOD	PORTION	CAL	PRO	VIT C	FOL	CA	IR
greens, raw; chopped	½ cup	21	2	22	–	90	1
roots, raw; cut up	½ cup	33	1	2	–	18	tr
witloof, raw	½ cup	7	tr	5	–	–	tr

CHILI

CANNED

FOOD	PORTION	CAL	PRO	VIT C	FOL	CA	IR
chili w/ beans	1 cup	286	15	4	–	119	9

FOOD	PORTION	CAL	PRO	VIT C	FOL	CA	IR
DRIED							
powder	1 tsp	8	tr	2	–	7	tr
TAKE-OUT							
con carne w/ beans	8.9 oz	254	25	2	30	67	5

CHINESE PRESERVING MELON

FOOD	PORTION	CAL	PRO	VIT C	FOL	CA	IR
cooked	½ cup	11	tr	9	–	16	tr

CHIPS

FOOD	PORTION	CAL	PRO	VIT C	FOL	CA	IR
POTATO							
potato	10 chips	105	1	8	9	5	tr
potato	1 oz	148	2	12	13	7	tr
sticks	1 oz pkg	148	2	13	11	5	1
sticks	½ cup	94	1	9	7	3	tr

CHITTERLINGS

FOOD	PORTION	CAL	PRO	VIT C	FOL	CA	IR
pork, raw	3 oz	213	–	–	–	18	–
pork; simmered	3 oz	258	24	0	–	23	3

CHIVES

FOOD	PORTION	CAL	PRO	VIT C	FOL	CA	IR
DRIED							
freeze-dried	1 tbsp	1	tr	1	–	2	tr
FRESH							
raw; chopped	1 tbsp	1	tr	2	3	2	tr

CHOCOLATE

FOOD	PORTION	CAL	PRO	VIT C	FOL	CA	IR
BAKING							
baking	1 oz	145	3	0	–	22	2
MIX							
powder	2–3 heaping tsp	75	1	tr	–	8	1
powder: as prep w/ whole milk	9 oz	226	9	3	12	300	1

FOOD	PORTION	CAL	PRO	VIT C	FOL	CA	IR
SYRUP							
chocolate	1 cup	653	6	1	12	42	6
chocolate	2 tbsp	82	1	tr	2	5	1
chocolate; as prep w/ whole milk	9 oz	232	9	2	14	297	1
CINNAMON							
ground	1 tsp	6	tr	1	–	28	1
CISCO							
FRESH							
raw	3 oz	84	16	–	–	–	–
SMOKED							
smoked	3 oz	151	14	–	2	22	tr
smoked	1 oz	50	5	–	1	7	tr
CLAMS							
CANNED							
liquid only	1 cup	6	1	–	–	31	–
liquid only	3 oz	2	tr	–	–	11	–
meat only	1 cup	236	41	–	158	148	45
meat only	3 oz	126	22	–	–	78	24
FRESH							
cooked	20 sm	133	23	–	–	83	25
cooked	3 oz	126	22	–	–	78	24
raw	3 oz	63	11	–	–	39	12
raw	9 lg	133	23	–	–	83	25
raw	20 sm	133	23	–	–	83	25
HOME RECIPE							
breaded & fried	3 oz	171	12	–	–	54	12
breaded & fried	20 sm	379	27	–	–	119	26
TAKE-OUT							
breaded & fried	¾ cup	451	13	0	9	21	3

FOOD	PORTION	CAL	PRO	VIT C	FOL	CA	IR
CLOVES							
ground	1 tsp	7	tr	2	–	14	tr
COCOA							
MIX							
powder	1 oz	102	3	1	0	93	tr
PREPARED							
home recipe	1 cup	218	9	2	12	298	1
hot cocoa	1 cup	218	9	2	12	298	1
mix w/ nutrasweet; as prep w/ water	7 oz	48	4	0	2	90	1
mix; as prep w/ water	7 oz	103	3	1	tr	96	tr
COCONUT							
coconut water	1 tbsp	3	tr	tr	–	4	tr
coconut water	1 cup	46	2	6	–	58	1
cream, canned	1 tbsp	36	1	–	–	0	tr
cream, canned	1 cup	568	8	–	–	4	2
dried, sweetened, flaked	7 oz. pkg	944	7	0	–	28	4
dried, sweetened, flaked	1 cup	351	2	0	–	10	1
dried, sweetened, flaked, canned	1 cup	341	3	–	–	11	1
dried, sweetened, shredded	7 oz pkg	997	6	1	–	30	4
dried, sweetened, shredded	1 cup	466	2	1	–	14	2
dried, toasted	1 oz	168	2	–	–	8	1
dried, unsweetened	1 oz	187	2	tr	3	7	1
milk, canned	1 tbsp	30	tr	tr	–	3	1
milk, canned	1 cup	445	5	2	–	40	7
milk, frozen	1 tbsp	30	tr	–	–	1	tr
milk, frozen	1 cup	486	4	–	–	11	2
raw; shredded	1 cup	283	3	3	21	12	2

FOOD	PORTION	CAL	PRO	VIT C	FOL	CA	IR
COD							
CANNED							
Atlantic	3 oz	89	19	1	–	18	tr
Atlantic	1 can (11 oz)	327	71	1	–	66	2
DRIED							
Atlantic	3 oz	246	53	3	–	136	2
FRESH							
Atlantic, raw	3 oz	70	15	1	–	13	tr
Atlantic; cooked	1 fillet (6.3 oz)	189	41	2	–	25	1
Atlantic; cooked	3 oz	89	19	1	–	12	tr
Pacific, raw	3 oz	70	15	–	–	6	tr
COFFEE							
INSTANT							
cappuccino mix; as prep w/ water	7 oz	62	tr	0	0	7	tr
decaffeinated	1 rounded tsp	4	tr	0	0	3	tr
decaffeinated; as prep w/ water	6 oz	4	tr	0	0	6	tr
french mix; as prep w/ water	7 oz	57	1	–	–	8	tr
mocha mix; as prep w/ water	7 oz	51	1	0	0	7	tr
regular	1 rounded tsp	4	tr	0	0	3	tr
regular w/ chicory	1 rounded tsp	6	tr	–	–	2	tr
regular w/ chicory; as prep w/ water	6 oz	6	tr	–	–	6	tr
regular; as prep w/ water	6 oz	4	tr	0	0	6	tr
REGULAR							
brewed	6 oz	4	tr	0	tr	3	1

FOOD	PORTION	CAL	PRO	VIT C	FOL	CA	IR
COFFEE SUBSTITUTES							
powder	1 tsp	9	tr	–	–	1	tr
powder; as prep w/ milk	6 oz	121	6	2	9	219	tr
powder; as prep w/ water	6 oz	9	tr	–	–	5	tr
COFFEE WHITENERS							
LIQUID nondairy, frzn	1 tbsp	20	tr	0	0	1	tr
POWDER nondairy	1 tsp	11	tr	0	0	tr	tr
COLLARDS							
FRESH cooked	½ cup	13	1	9	4	74	tr
raw; chopped	½ cup	18	1	22	2	109	1
FROZEN chopped; cooked	½ cup	31	3	23	65	179	1
COOKIES							
HOME RECIPE chocolate chip	4 (1½ oz)	185	2	0	–	13	1
peanut butter	4 (1.7 oz)	245	4	0	–	21	1
shortbread	2 (1 oz)	145	2	tr	–	6	1
READY-TO-EAT animal crackers	1 box (2.4 oz)	299	4	tr	22	11	1
chocolate sandwich	4 (1.4 oz)	195	2	0	–	12	1
chocolate chip	4 (1½ oz)	180	2	tr	–	13	1
chocolate chip	1 box (1.9 oz)	233	3	tr	16	20	1
fig bars	4 (2 oz)	210	2	tr	–	40	1
graham	2 squares	60	1	0	–	6	tr

FOOD	PORTION	CAL	PRO	VIT C	FOL	CA	IR
oatmeal raisin	4 (1.8 oz)	245	3	0	–	18	1
shortbread	4 (1 oz)	155	2	0	–	13	1
vanilla sandwich	4 (1.4 oz)	195	2	0	–	12	1
vanilla wafers	10 (1¼ oz)	185	2	0	–	16	1
REFRIGERATED chocolate chip	4 (1.7 oz)	225	2	0	–	13	1
sugar	4 (1.7 oz)	235	2	0	–	50	1

CORIANDER

FOOD	PORTION	CAL	PRO	VIT C	FOL	CA	IR
leaf, dried	1 tsp	2	tr	3	–	7	tr
seed	1 tsp	5	tr	–	–	13	tr
FRESH coriander	¼ cup	1	tr	tr	–	4	tr

CORN

FOOD	PORTION	CAL	PRO	VIT C	FOL	CA	IR
CANNED cream style	½ cup	93	2	6	57	4	tr
w/ red & green peppers	½ cup	86	3	10	–	5	1
white	½ cup	66	2	–	–	–	1
yellow	½ cup	66	2	–	–	–	1
FRESH on-the-cob w/ butter; cooked	1 ear	155	4	7	44	5	tr
white, raw	½ cup	66	2	5	35	2	tr
white; cooked	½ cup	89	3	5	38	2	1
yellow, raw	½ cup	66	2	5	35	2	tr
yellow, raw	1 ear (3 oz)	77	3	6	41	2	tr
yellow; cooked	1 ear (2.7 oz)	83	3	5	36	2	tr
yellow; cooked	½ cup	89	3	5	38	2	1

FOOD	PORTION	CAL	PRO	VIT C	FOL	CA	IR
FROZEN							
cooked	½ cup	67	2	2	19	2	tr
on-the-cob; cooked	1 ear (2.2 oz)	59	2	3	19	2	tr

CORNMEAL

FOOD	PORTION	CAL	PRO	VIT C	FOL	CA	IR
corn grits, uncooked	1 cup	579	14	–	7	3	6
corn grits; cooked	1 cup	146	4	–	1	1	2
degermed	1 cup	506	12	0	66	7	6
self-rising, degermed	1 cup	489	12	0	43	482	7
whole grain	1 cup	442	10	0	–	7	4

CORNSTARCH

FOOD	PORTION	CAL	PRO	VIT C	FOL	CA	IR
cornstarch	1 cup	164	tr	0	–	1	tr

COTTAGE CHEESE

FOOD	PORTION	CAL	PRO	VIT C	FOL	CA	IR
REDUCED CALORIE							
lowfat, 1%	4 oz	82	14	tr	14	69	tr
lowfat, 1%	1 cup	164	28	tr	28	138	tr
lowfat, 2%	4 oz	101	16	tr	15	77	tr
lowfat, 2%	1 cup	203	31	tr	30	155	tr
REGULAR							
creamed	4 oz	117	14	tr	14	68	tr
creamed	1 cup	217	26	tr	26	126	tr
dry curd	1 cup	123	25	0	21	46	tr
dry curd	4 oz	96	20	0	17	36	tr

COTTONSEED

FOOD	PORTION	CAL	PRO	VIT C	FOL	CA	IR
kernals, roasted	1 tbsp	51	3	1	–	10	1

COUSCOUS

FOOD	PORTION	CAL	PRO	VIT C	FOL	CA	IR
cooked	½ cup	101	3	–	13	8	tr
dry	½ cup	346	12	0	16	22	1

FOOD	PORTION	CAL	PRO	VIT C	FOL	CA	IR
CANNED							
common	1 cup	184	11	7	123	48	2
common w/ pork	½ cup	199	7	1	–	21	3
DRIED							
catjang, raw	1 cup	572	20	3	1067	141	17
catjang; cooked	1 cup	200	14	1	242	44	5
common, raw	1 cup	562	39	3	1056	183	14
common; cooked	1 cup	198	13	1	356	42	4
FRESH							
leafy tips, raw; chopped	1 cup	10	1	13	–	23	1
leafy tips; chopped, cooked	1 cup	12	2	10	–	36	1
FROZEN							
cooked	½ cup	112	7	2	120	20	2

CRAB

FOOD	PORTION	CAL	PRO	VIT C	FOL	CA	IR
CANNED							
blue	3 oz	84	17	–	–	86	1
blue	1 cup	133	28	–	–	137	1
FRESH							
Alaska king, raw	1 leg (6 oz)	144	32	–	–	80	1
alaska king, raw	3 oz	71	16	–	–	39	1
alaska king; cooked	1 leg (4.7 oz)	129	26	–	–	80	1
alaska king; cooked	3 oz	82	16	–	–	50	1
blue, raw	3 oz	74	15	–	–	76	1
blue, raw	1 crab (.7 oz)	18	4	–	–	19	tr
blue: cooked	3 oz	87	17	–	–	88	1
blue; cooked	1 cup	138	27	–	–	140	1
dungeness, raw	1 crab (5.7 oz)	140	28	–	–	75	1

FOOD	PORTION	CAL	PRO	VIT C	FOL	CA	IR
dungeness, raw	3 oz	73	15	–	–	39	tr
queen, raw	3 oz	76	16	–	–	22	–
READY-TO-USE							
crab cakes	1 cake (2.1 oz)	93	12	–	–	63	1
TAKE-OUT							
baked	1 (2 oz)	88	16	2	20	228	tr
cake	1 (3.8 oz)	290	20	tr	17	367	2
soft-shell; fried	1 (4.4 oz)	334	11	tr	20	55	2

CRACKERS

FOOD	PORTION	CAL	PRO	VIT C	FOL	CA	IR
cheese	10 (⅓ oz)	50	1	0	–	11	tr
crispbread	3½ oz	317	9	0	tr	55	5
melba toast, plain	1	20	1	0	–	6	tr
peanut butter sandwich	1 (⅓ oz)	40	1	0	–	7	tr
saltines	4	50	1	0	–	3	1
zwieback	3½ oz	374	9	–	–	42	2

CRANBERRIES

FOOD	PORTION	CAL	PRO	VIT C	FOL	CA	IR
CANNED							
cranberry sauce, sweetened	½ cup	209	tr	3	–	5	tr
FRESH							
chopped	1 cup	54	tr	15	2	8	tr
JUICE							
cranberry juice cocktail	1 cup	147	tr	108	1	8	tr
cranberry juice cocktail	6 oz	108	0	67	1	7	tr
cranberry juice cocktail, frzn	12 oz	821	tr	148	0	48	1
cranberry juice cocktail, frzn; as prep	6 oz	102	0	18	0	9	tr
low calorie cranberry juice cocktail	6 oz	33	0	57	–	16	tr

FOOD	PORTION	CAL	PRO	VIT C	FOL	CA	IR
CRANBERRY BEANS							
CANNED							
cranberry beans	1 cup	216	14	2	201	67	4
DRIED							
cooked	1 cup	240	17	0	366	44	4
raw	1 cup	652	45	0	1179	248	10
CRAYFISH							
FRESH							
cooked	3 oz	97	20	3	–	26	3
raw	3 oz	76	16	3	–	20	2
raw	8	24	5	1	–	6	1
CREAM							
LIQUID							
half & half	1 tbsp	20	tr	tr	tr	16	tr
half & half	1 cup	315	7	2	6	254	tr
heavy whipping	1 tbsp	52	tr	tr	1	10	tr
light whipping	1 tbsp	44	tr	tr	1	10	tr
light, coffee	1 tbsp	29	tr	tr	tr	14	tr
light, coffee	1 cup	496	6	2	6	14	tr
WHIPPED							
heavy whipping	1 cup	411	5	1	9	77	tr
light whipping	1 cup	345	5	1	9	83	tr
CREAM CHEESE							
NEUFCHATEL							
neufchatel	1 oz	74	3	0	3	21	tr
neufchatel	1 pkg (3 oz)	221	8	0	10	64	tr
REGULAR							
cream cheese	1 oz	99	2	0	4	23	tr
cream cheese	1 pkg (3 oz)	297	6	0	11	68	1

FOOD	PORTION	CAL	PRO	VIT C	FOL	CA	IR
CRESS							
FRESH							
garden, raw	½ cup	8	tr	17	–	20	tr
garden; cooked	½ cup	16	1	16	–	41	1
CROAKER							
Atlantic, raw	3 oz	89	15	–	–	13	tr
Atlantic; breaded & fried	3 oz	188	15	–	–	27	1
CROISSANT							
croissant	1 (2 oz)	235	5	0	–	20	2
TAKE-OUT							
w/ egg & cheese	1	369	13	tr	36	244	2
w/ egg, cheese & bacon	1	413	16	2	35	151	2
w/ egg, cheese & ham	1	475	19	11	36	144	2
w/ egg, cheese & sausage	1	524	20	tr	38	144	3
CUCUMBER							
FRESH							
raw	1 (11 oz)	39	2	14	42	42	1
raw; sliced	½ cup	7	tr	2	7	7	tr
CUMIN							
seed	1 tsp	8	tr	tr	–	20	1
CURRANTS							
DRIED							
zante	½ cup	204	3	3	7	62	2
FRESH							
black	½ cup	36	1	101	–	31	1
JUICE							
black currant nectar	3½ oz	55	tr	30	tr	15	tr
red currant nectar	3½ oz	54	tr	6	tr	7	tr

FOOD	PORTION	CAL	PRO	VIT C	FOL	CA	IR
CUSK							
FRESH							
raw	3 oz	74	–	–	–	9	1
CUSTARD							
baked	1 cup	305	14	1	–	297	1
CUTTLEFISH							
FRESH							
raw	3 oz	67	14	–	5	77	5
DANDELION GREENS							
cooked	½ cup	17	1	9	–	73	1
raw; chopped	½ cup	13	1	10	–	52	1
DANISH PASTRY							
cheese	1 (3 oz)	353	6	3	15	70	2
cinnamon	1 (3 oz)	349	5	3	14	37	2
fruit	1 (2.3 oz)	235	4	tr	–	17	1
fruit	1 (3.3 oz)	335	5	2	15	22	1
plain	1 (2 oz)	220	4	tr	–	60	1
plain ring	1 (12 oz)	1305	21	tr	–	360	7
DATES							
DRIED							
chopped	1 cup	489	4	0	22	58	2
whole	10	228	2	0	10	27	1
DILL							
seed	1 tsp	6	tr	–	–	32	tr
weed, dried	1 tsp	3	tr	–	–	18	tr

FOOD	PORTION	CAL	PRO	VIT C	FOL	CA	IR
DOCK							
FRESH							
cooked	3½ oz	20	2	26	–	38	2
raw; chopped	½ cup	15	1	32	–	29	2
DOGFISH							
raw	3½ oz	193	13	–	–	5	1
DOLPHINFISH							
FRESH							
raw	3 oz	73	16	–	–	–	1
DOUGHNUTS							
cake type	1 (1.8 oz)	210	3	tr	–	22	1
glazed	1 (2 oz)	235	4	0	–	17	1
DRINK MIXER							
whiskey sour mix	2 oz	55	0	2	0	1	tr
DRUM							
FRESH							
freshwater, raw	3 oz	101	15	–	–	51	1
DUCK							
w/ skin, raw	½ duck (1.4 lbs)	2561	73	18	81	67	15
w/ skin; roasted	6 oz	583	33	0	11	20	5
w/ skin; roasted	½ duck (13.4 oz)	1287	73	0	25	43	10
w/o skin, raw	4.8 oz	180	25	8	34	15	3
w/o skin; roasted	3.5 oz	201	23	0	10	12	3
w/o skin; roasted	½ duck (7.8 oz)	445	52	0	22	26	6
wild breast w/o skin, raw	½ breast (2.9 oz)	102	16	5	–	3	4

FOOD	PORTION	CAL	PRO	VIT C	FOL	CA	IR
wild w/ skin, raw	½ duck (9.5 oz)	571	47	14	–	12	11

DURIAN

fresh	3½ oz	141	3	42	–	12	1

EEL

FRESH

cooked	3 oz	200	20	–	–	22	1
cooked	1 fillet (5.6 oz)	375	38	–	–	41	1
raw	3 oz	156	16	–	–	17	tr

EGG

CHICKEN

fried w/ margarine	1	91	6	0	18	25	1
frozen	1	75	6	0	23	25	1
frozen	1 cup	363	30	0	114	120	4
hard cooked	1	77	6	0	22	25	1
hard cooked; chopped	1 cup	210	17	0	60	68	2
poached	1	74	6	0	18	25	1
raw	1	75	6	0	23	25	1
raw	1 cup	363	30	0	114	120	4
scrambled w/ whole milk & margarine	1	101	7	0	18	44	1
scrambled w/ whole milk & margarine	1 cup	365	24	1	66	157	3
scrambled, plain	2	200	13	3	52	54	2
white only	1	17	4	0	1	2	tr
white only	1 cup	121	26	0	7	15	tr
yolk, raw	1 cup	870	41	0	354	333	9
yolk, raw	1	59	3	0	24	23	1

FOOD	PORTION	CAL	PRO	VIT C	FOL	CA	IR
OTHER POULTRY							
duck, raw	1	130	9	0	56	45	3
goose, raw	1	267	20	0	–	–	–
quail, raw	1	14	1	0	–	6	tr
turkey, raw	1	135	9	0	–	78	3
EGG DISHES							
TAKE-OUT							
sandwich w/ cheese, ham	1	348	19	3	43	212	3
sandwich w/ cheese	1	340	16	2	36	225	3
EGG SUBSTITUTES							
frozen	¼ cup	96	7	–	–	44	1
frozen	1 cup	384	27	–	–	175	5
liquid	1½ oz	40	6	0	–	25	1
liquid	1 cup	211	30	0	–	133	5
powder	0.7 oz	88	11	tr	–	32	1
powder	0.35 oz	44	5	tr	–	32	tr
EGGNOG							
eggnog	1 cup	342	10	4	2	330	1
eggnog	1 qt	1368	39	15	9	1321	2
eggnog flavor mix; as prep w/ milk	9 oz	260	8	2	12	291	tr
EGGPLANT							
FRESH							
cubed, cooked	½ cup	13	tr	1	7	3	tr
raw, cut up	½ cup	11	tr	1	7	15	tr
ELDERBERRIES							
elderberries	1 cup	105	1	52	–	55	2
JUICE							
elderberry	3½ oz	38	2	26	6	5	–

FOOD	PORTION	CAL	PRO	VIT C	FOL	CA	IR
ELK							
raw	1 oz	32	7	–	–	1	1
roasted	3 oz	124	26	–	–	4	3
ENDIVE							
FRESH							
fresh	3½ oz	9	2	–	tr	54	1
raw; chopped	½ cup	4	tr	2	36	13	tr
ENGLISH MUFFIN							
plain; toasted	1	140	5	0	–	96	2
TAKE-OUT							
w/ butter	1	189	5	tr	17	103	2
w/ cheese & sausage	1	394	15	1	18	168	2
w/ egg, cheese & bacon	1	487	22	1	54	196	3
w/ egg, cheese & canadian bacon	1	383	20	1	44	207	3
EPPAW							
raw	½ cup	75	2	7	–	55	1
FALAFEL							
falafel	1 (1.2 oz)	57	2	tr	13	9	1
falafel	3 (1.8 oz)	170	7	1	40	27	2
FAT							
beef suet, raw	1 oz	242	tr	–	–	–	–
beef tallow	1 tbsp	115	0	–	–	–	–
beef, raw	1 oz	191	2	0	1	3	tr
beef; cooked	1 oz	193	3	0	1	4	tr
chicken	1 cup	1846	0	–	–	–	–
chicken	1 tbsp	115	0	–	–	–	–
chicken, raw	1 oz	201	1	0	0	2	tr
cocoa butter	1 tbsp	120	0	–	–	–	–

FOOD	PORTION	CAL	PRO	VIT C	FOL	CA	IR
duck	1 tbsp	115	0	–	–	–	–
goose	1 tbsp	115	0	–	–	–	–
lamb, new zealand, raw	1 oz	182	2	–	–	6	tr
lard	1 cup	1849	0	–	–	tr	–
lard	1 tbsp	115	0	–	–	tr	–
nutmeg butter	1 tbsp	120	0	–	–	–	–
pork backfat	1 oz	230	–	–	–	1	–
pork, cured, uncooked	1 oz	164	–	–	–	1	–
pork, cured; roasted	1 oz	167	–	–	–	2	–
pork; cooked	1 oz	200	2	0	tr	1	tr
salt pork	1 oz	212	23	–	0	2	tr
shortening	1 tbsp	113	0	–	–	–	–
turkey	1 tbsp	115	0	–	–	–	–
ucuhuba butter	1 tbsp	120	0	–	–	–	–

FENNEL

FOOD	PORTION	CAL	PRO	VIT C	FOL	CA	IR
seed	1 tsp	7	tr	–	–	24	tr

FENUGREEK

FOOD	PORTION	CAL	PRO	VIT C	FOL	CA	IR
seed	1 tsp	12	1	tr	2	6	1

FIGS

FOOD	PORTION	CAL	PRO	VIT C	FOL	CA	IR
CANNED							
in heavy syrup	3	75	tr	1	–	23	tr
in light syrup	3	58	tr	1	–	23	tr
water pack	3	42	tr	1	–	22	tr
DRIED							
cooked	½ cup	140	2	6	1	79	1
whole	10	477	6	2	14	269	4
FRESH							
fig	1 med	50	tr	1	–	18	tr

FOOD	PORTION	CAL	PRO	VIT C	FOL	CA	IR
FILBERTS							
dried, unblanched	1 oz	179	4	tr	20	53	1
dried, blanched	1 oz	191	4	–	–	55	1
dry roasted, unblanched	1 oz	188	3	–	–	55	1
oil roasted, unblanched	1 oz	187	4	–	–	56	1
FISH							
FROZEN							
breaded fillet; as prep	1 (2 oz)	155	9	–	10	11	tr
sticks; as prep	1 stick (1 oz)	76	4	–	5	6	tr
TAKE-OUT							
sandwich w/ tartar sauce	1	431	17	3	44	84	3
sandwich w/ tartar sauce, cheese	1	524	21	3	32	185	4
FLATFISH							
FRESH							
cooked	1 fillet (4.5 oz)	148	31	–	–	23	tr
cooked	3 oz	99	21	–	–	16	tr
raw	3 oz	78	16	–	–	15	tr
TAKE-OUT							
battered & fried	3.2 oz	211	13	0	51	17	2
breaded & fried	3.2 oz	211	13	0	51	17	2
FLOUR							
corn, masa	1 cup	416	11	0	28	161	8
corn, whole grain	1 cup	422	8	0	30	8	3
cottonseed, lowfat	1 oz	94	14	1	–	135	4
peanut, defatted	1 cup	196	31	–	–	84	1
peanut, defatted	1 oz	92	15	0	70	39	1
peanut, lowfat	1 oz	120	9	–	–	36	1

FOOD	PORTION	CAL	PRO	VIT C	FOL	CA	IR
peanut, lowfat	1 cup	257	20	–	–	78	3
potato	1 cup	628	14	34	–	59	31
rice, brown	1 cup	574	11	0	25	18	3
rice, white	1 cup	578	9	0	6	16	tr
rye, dark	1 cup	415	18	0	77	72	8
rye, light	1 cup	374	9	0	23	21	2
rye, medium	1 cup	361	10	0	20	24	2
sesame, lowfat	1 oz	95	14	–	8	42	4
triticale, whole grain	1 cup	440	17	0	96	45	3
white, all-purpose	1 cup	455	13	0	33	18	6
white, bread	1 cup	495	16	0	40	21	6
white, cake	1 cup	395	9	0	21	16	8
white, self-rising	1 cup	442	12	0	53	422	6
whole wheat	1 cup	407	16	0	52	40	5

FRENCH BEANS

DRIED

cooked	1 cup	228	12	2	132	111	2
raw	1 cup	631	35	8	733	342	6

FRENCH TOAST

HOME RECIPE

french toast	1 slice	155	6	tr	–	72	1

TAKE-OUT

w/ butter	2 slices	356	10	tr	30	73	2

FRUIT DRINKS

FROZEN

citrus juice drink	12 oz	684	5	403	30	106	17
citrus juice drink; as prep	1 cup	114	1	67	5	21	3
fruit punch	1 can (12 oz)	678	1	650	14	33	1

FOOD	PORTION	CAL	PRO	VIT C	FOL	CA	IR
fruit punch; as prep w/ water	1 cup	113	tr	108	2	9	tr
lemonade	1 can (6 oz)	397	1	39	22	15	2
lemonade; as prep w/ water	1 cup	100	tr	10	6	8	tr
limeade	1 can (6 oz)	408	tr	–	–	11	tr
limeade; as prep w/ water	1 cup	102	tr	–	–	7	tr
MIX							
fruit punch; as prep w/ water	9 oz	97	tr	31	tr	41	tr
lemonade powder w/ nutrasweet; as prep w/ water	1 pitcher (67 oz)	40	tr	47	0	408	1
lemonade powder; as prep w/ water	9 oz	113	0	34	0	29	tr
READY-TO-USE							
cranberry apricot drink	6 oz	118	0	0	–	17	tr
cranberry apple drink	6 oz	123	tr	–	–	13	tr
fruit punch	6 oz	87	tr	55	2	14	tr
orange & apricot drink	1 cup	128	1	50	–	13	tr
orange-grapefruit juice	1 cup	107	1	72	–	21	1
pineapple & grapefruit drink	1 cup	117	1	115	26	18	1
pineapple & orange drink	1 cup	125	3	56	27	13	1

FRUIT MIXED

FOOD	PORTION	CAL	PRO	VIT C	FOL	CA	IR
CANNED							
fruit cocktail in heavy syrup	½ cup	93	1	2	–	8	tr
fruit cocktail water pack	½ cup	40	1	3	–	6	tr
fruit cocktail juice pack	½ cup	56	1	3	–	10	tr
fruit salad juice pack	½ cup	62	1	4	–	14	tr

FOOD	PORTION	CAL	PRO	VIT C	FOL	CA	IR
fruit salad juice pack	½ cup	62	1	4	–	14	tr
fruit salad water pack	½ cup	37	tr	2	–	8	tr
fruit salad in heavy syrup	½ cup	94	tr	3	–	8	tr
fruit salad in light syrup	½ cup	73	tr	3	–	8	tr
mixed fruit in heavy syrup	½ cup	92	tr	88	–	1	tr
tropical fruit salad in heavy syrup	½ cup	110	1	22	–	17	1
DRIED mixed	11 oz pkg	712	7	11	–	110	8
FROZEN mixed fruit sweetened	1 cup	245	4	188	–	18	1

GARLIC

FOOD	PORTION	CAL	PRO	VIT C	FOL	CA	IR
powder	1 tsp	9	tr	–	–	2	tr
FRESH clove	1	4	tr	1	tr	5	tr

GEFILTE FISH

FOOD	PORTION	CAL	PRO	VIT C	FOL	CA	IR
READY-TO-USE sweet recipe	1 piece (1.5 oz)	35	4	–	1	10	1

GELATIN

FOOD	PORTION	CAL	PRO	VIT C	FOL	CA	IR
MIX fruit flavored; as prep	½ cup	70	2	0	–	2	tr
low calorie	½ cup	8	2	0	0	tr	tr

GIBLETS

FOOD	PORTION	CAL	PRO	VIT C	FOL	CA	IR
capon, raw	4 oz	150	21	21	453	11	7
capon; simmered	1 cup (5 oz)	238	38	13	601	19	10
chicken; floured, fried	1 cup (5 oz)	402	47	13	550	26	15
chicken; simmered	1 cup (5 oz)	228	37	12	545	18	9

FOOD	PORTION	CAL	PRO	VIT C	FOL	CA	IR
chicken; raw	2.6 oz	93	13	12	259	7	4
turkey, raw	8.6 oz	314	47	9	834	20	17
turkey; simmered	1 cup (5 oz)	243	39	3	501	18	10

GINGER

FOOD	PORTION	CAL	PRO	VIT C	FOL	CA	IR
ground	1 tsp	6	tr	–	–	2	tr
root, fresh	5 slices	8	tr	1	–	2	tr
root, fresh	¼ cup	17	tr	1	–	4	tr

GINKGO NUTS

FOOD	PORTION	CAL	PRO	VIT C	FOL	CA	IR
canned	1 oz	32	1	–	–	1	tr
dried	1 oz	99	3	8	–	6	tr
raw	1 oz	52	1	4	–	1	tr

GIZZARDS

FOOD	PORTION	CAL	PRO	VIT C	FOL	CA	IR
chicken; simmered	1 cup (5 oz)	222	5	2	77	14	6
chicken; raw	1 (1.3 oz)	41	7	1	19	3	1
turkey, raw	1 (4 oz)	133	22	4	59	10	4
turkey; simmered	1 cup (5 oz)	236	43	2	75	22	8

GOAT

FOOD	PORTION	CAL	PRO	VIT C	FOL	CA	IR
raw	1 oz	31	6	–	1	4	1
roasted	3 oz	122	23	–	5	15	3

GOOSE

FRESH

FOOD	PORTION	CAL	PRO	VIT C	FOL	CA	IR
w/ skin, raw	½ goose (2.9 lb)	4893	209	–	57	158	33
w/ skin; roasted	6.6 oz	574	47	0	4	25	5
w/ skin; roasted	½ goose (1.7 lbs)	2362	195	0	17	104	22

FOOD	PORTION	CAL	PRO	VIT C	FOL	CA	IR
w/o skin; roasted	5 oz	340	41	–	–	20	4
w/o skin; roasted	½ goose (1.3 lbs)	1406	171	–	–	84	17

GOOSEBERRIES

fresh	1 cup	67	1	42	–	38	tr
CANNED in light syrup	½ cup	93	1	13	4	20	tr

GRAPEFRUIT

juice pack	½ cup	46	1	42	–	19	tr
unsweetened	1 cup	93	1	72	26	18	1
water pack	½ cup	44	1	27	11	18	1
FRESH pink	½	37	1	47	15	13	tr
pink sections	1 cup	69	1	88	28	25	tr
red	½	37	1	47	15	13	tr
red sections	1 cup	69	1	88	28	25	tr
white	½	39	1	39	12	17	tr
white sections	1 cup	76	2	77	23	28	tr
JUICE fresh	1 cup	96	1	94	–	22	tr
frzn; as prep	1 cup	102	1	83	9	19	tr
frzn; not prep	6 oz	302	4	248	26	18	1
sweetened	1 cup	116	1	67	26	20	1

GRAPES

CANNED thompson seedless in heavy syrup	½ cup	94	1	1	–	13	1
thompson seedless water pack	½ cup	48	1	1	–	13	1

FOOD	PORTION	CAL	PRO	VIT C	FOL	CA	IR
FRESH							
grapes	10	36	tr	5	2	5	tr
JUICE							
bottled	1 cup	155	1	tr	7	22	1
frzn sweetened; not prep	6 oz	386	1	180	9	28	1
frzn, sweetened; as prep	1 cup	128	tr	60	3	9	tr
grape drink	6 oz	84	0	64	1	–	tr
GRAVY							
CANNED							
au jus	1 cup	38	3	2	–	10	1
beef	1 cup	124	9	0	–	14	2
chicken	1 cup	189	5	0	–	48	1
mushroom	1 cup	120	3	0	–	17	2
turkey	1 cup	122	6	0	–	10	2
DRY							
au jus; as prep	1 cup	19	1	–	–	11	–
brown; as prep	1 cup	9	tr	–	–	7	tr
chicken; as prep	1 cup	83	3	–	–	39	–
mushroom; as prep	1 cup	70	2	–	–	49	–
pork; as prep	1 cup	76	2	–	–	32	–
turkey; as prep	1 cup	87	3	–	–	50	–
GREAT NORTHERN BEANS							
CANNED							
great northern	1 cup	300	19	3	213	139	4
DRIED							
cooked	1 cup	210	15	2	181	121	4
raw	1 cup	621	40	10	882	320	10
GROUNDCHERRIES							
fresh	½ cup	37	1	8	–	6	1

FOOD	PORTION	CAL	PRO	VIT C	FOL	CA	IR
GROUPER							
FRESH							
cooked	1 fillet (7.1 oz)	238	50	–	–	42	2
cooked	3 oz	100	21	–	–	18	1
raw	3 oz	78	16	–	–	23	1
GUAVA							
guava sauce	½ cup	43	tr	174	–	8	tr
FRESH							
guava	1	45	1	165	–	18	tr
GUINEA HEN							
w/ skin, raw	½ hen (12.1 oz)	545	81	–	–	–	–
w/o skin, raw	½ hen (9.3 oz)	292	55	–	–	–	–
HADDOCK							
cooked	1 fillet (5.3 oz)	168	36	–	–	64	2
cooked	3 oz	95	21	–	–	36	1
raw	3 oz	74	16	–	–	28	1
SMOKED							
smoked	3 oz	99	21	–	–	41	1
smoked	1 oz	33	7	–	–	14	tr
HAKE							
raw	3½ oz	84	17	–	–	41	–
HALIBUT							
FRESH							
Atlantic & Pacific, raw	3 oz	93	18	–	–	40	1
Atlantic & Pacific; cooked	3 oz	119	23	–	–	51	1

FOOD	PORTION	CAL	PRO	VIT C	FOL	CA	IR
Atlantic & Pacific; cooked	½ fillet (5.6 oz)	223	42	–	–	95	2
Greenland, raw	3 oz	158	12	–	1	3	1

HAM

FOOD	PORTION	CAL	PRO	VIT C	FOL	CA	IR
canned (13% fat); roasted	3 oz	192	17	12	4	7	1
canned, extra lean (4% fat)	3 oz	116	18	23	5	5	1
chopped	1 oz	65	5	6	0	2	tr
chopped, canned	1 oz	68	5	0	–	2	tr
ham & cheese loaf	1 oz	73	9	14	–	33	1
ham & cheese spread	1 tbsp	37	2	1	–	33	tr
ham & cheese spread	1 oz	69	5	2	–	62	tr
ham salad spread	1 tbsp	32	1	1	–	1	tr
ham salad spread	1 oz	61	2	2	–	2	tr
minced	1 oz	75	5	8	–	3	tr
sliced, extra lean (5% fat)	1 oz	37	5	7	1	2	tr
sliced, regular (11% fat)	1 oz	52	5	8	1	2	tr
steak, boneless, extra lean	1 oz	35	6	9	1	1	tr

HAM DISHES

TAKE-OUT

FOOD	PORTION	CAL	PRO	VIT C	FOL	CA	IR
sandwich w/ cheese	1	353	21	3	71	130	3

HAMBURGER

TAKE-OUT

FOOD	PORTION	CAL	PRO	VIT C	FOL	CA	IR
double patty w/ bun, cheese	1 reg	457	28	0	29	232	3
double patty w/ bun	1 reg	544	30	0	38	87	5
double patty w/ bun, catsup, mayonnaise, mustard, pickle, onion, tomato	1 lg	540	34	1	27	102	6

FOOD	PORTION	CAL	PRO	VIT C	FOL	CA	IR
double patty w/ bun, catsup, mustard, pickle, onion	1 reg	576	32	1	45	92	6
double patty w/ bun, cheese, catsup, mustard, mayonnaise, pickle, tomato	1 lg	706	38	tr	48	240	6
double patty w/ bun, cheese, catsup, pickle, mayonnaise, onion, tomato	1 reg	416	21	2	23	171	3
double patty w/ double bun, catsup, pickle, mayonnaise, onion, tomato	1 reg	649	30	3	34	169	5
double patty w/ double bun, cheese	1 reg	461	22	0	36	224	4
single patty w/ bun	1 reg	275	12	0	25	63	2
single patty w/ bun	1 lg	400	23	0	32	74	4
single patty w/ bun, catsup, mayonnaise, mustard, pickle, onion, tomato	1 reg	279	13	2	18	63	3
single patty w/ bun, cheese	1 reg	320	15	0	26	140	2
single patty w/ bun, cheese	1 lg	608	30	32	38	91	5
single patty w/ bun, cheese, bacon, catsup, mustard, pickle, onion	1 lg	609	32	2	33	162	5
single patty w/ bun, cheese, ham, catsup, mayonnaise, pickle, tomato	1 lg	745	40	7	50	301	5
triple patty w/ bun, catsup, mustard, pickle	1 lg	693	50	1	31	65	8

FOOD	PORTION	CAL	PRO	VIT C	FOL	CA	IR
triple patty w/ bun, cheese	1 lg	769	56	3	51	282	8

HEART

beef; simmered	3 oz	148	24	1	2	5	6
chicken; simmered	1 cup (5 oz)	268	11	3	116	27	13
chicken; raw	1 (⅕ oz)	9	1	tr	4	1	tr
lamb; braised	3 oz	158	21	6	2	12	5
turkey, raw	1 (1 oz)	41	5	1	21	3	1
turkey; simmered	1 cup (5 oz)	257	39	3	114	19	10
veal; braised	3 oz	158	25	–	–	7	4

HERBS/SPICES

DRIED

curry powder	1 tsp	6	tr	tr	–	10	1
poultry seasoning	1 tsp	5	tr	tr	–	15	1
pumpkin pie spice	1 tsp	6	tr	tr	–	12	tr

HERRING

FRESH

Atlantic, raw	3 oz	134	15	1	–	49	1
Atlantic; cooked	1 fillet (5 oz)	290	33	1	–	105	2
Atlantic; cooked	3 oz	172	20	1	–	63	1
Pacific, raw	3 oz	166	14	–	–	–	1
READY-TO-USE Atlantic, kippered	1 fillet (1.4 oz)	87	10	tr	–	33	1
Atlantic, pickled	½ oz	39	2	–	tr	12	tr

HICKORY NUTS

dried	1 oz	187	4	–	–	17	1

FOOD	PORTION	CAL	PRO	VIT C	FOL	CA	IR

HOMINY

CANNED

FOOD	PORTION	CAL	PRO	VIT C	FOL	CA	IR
canned	½ cup	57	1	0	1	8	tr
honey	1 cup	1030	1	3	–	17	2
honey	1 tbsp	65	tr	tr	–	1	tr

HONEYDEW

FOOD	PORTION	CAL	PRO	VIT C	FOL	CA	IR
cubed	1 cup	60	1	42	–	10	tr
fresh	⅒	46	1	32	–	8	tr

HORSE

FOOD	PORTION	CAL	PRO	VIT C	FOL	CA	IR
raw	1 oz	38	6	0	–	2	1
roasted	3 oz	149	24	2	–	7	4

HOT DOG

CHICKEN

FOOD	PORTION	CAL	PRO	VIT C	FOL	CA	IR
chicken	1 (1.5 oz)	116	6	–	–	43	1

MEAT

FOOD	PORTION	CAL	PRO	VIT C	FOL	CA	IR
beef	1 (2 oz)	184	6	14	2	7	1
beef	1 (1.6 oz)	145	5	11	2	6	1
beef & pork	1 (2 oz)	183	6	15	2	6	1
beef & pork	1 (1.6 oz)	144	5	12	2	6	1

TAKE-OUT

FOOD	PORTION	CAL	PRO	VIT C	FOL	CA	IR
corndog	1	460	17	0	60	101	6
w/ bun, chili	1	297	14	3	50	19	3
w/ bun, plain	1	242	10	tr	30	24	2

TURKEY

FOOD	PORTION	CAL	PRO	VIT C	FOL	CA	IR
turkey	1 (1.5 oz)	102	6	–	–	48	1

HUMMUS

FOOD	PORTION	CAL	PRO	VIT C	FOL	CA	IR
hummus	⅓ cup	140	4	6	49	41	1
hummus	1 cup	420	12	19	146	124	4

FOOD	PORTION	CAL	PRO	VIT C	FOL	CA	IR
HYACINTH BEANS							
DRIED							
cooked	1 cup	228	16	0	–	77	9
raw	1 cup	723	50	0	–	273	11
ICE CREAM AND FROZEN DESSERTS							
french vanilla, soft serve	1 cup	377	7	1	9	236	tr
french vanilla, soft serve	½ gal	3014	56	7	73	1886	3
orange sherbet	1 cup	270	2	4	14	103	tr
orange sherbet	½ gal	2158	17	31	111	827	2
vanilla ice milk, soft serve	1 cup	223	8	1	5	274	tr
vanilla ice milk, soft serve	½ gal	1787	64	9	38	2195	2
vanilla ice milk	1 cup	184	5	1	3	176	tr
vanilla ice milk	½ gal	1469	41	6	24	1409	1
vanilla, 10% fat	1 cup	269	5	1	3	176	tr
vanilla, 10% fat	½ gal	2153	38	6	22	1406	1
vanilla, 16% fat	1 cup	349	4	1	2	151	tr
vanilla, 16% fat	½ gal	2805	33	5	19	1213	1
TAKE-OUT							
cone, vanilla, ice milk, soft serve	1 (4.6 oz)	164	4	1	5	153	tr
sundae, caramel	1 (5.4 oz)	303	7	3	12	189	tr
sundae, hot fudge	1 (5.4 oz)	284	6	2	9	207	tr
sundae, strawberry	1 (5.4 oz)	269	6	2	18	161	tr
JACKFRUIT							
fresh	3½ oz	70	1	9	–	27	1

FOOD	PORTION	CAL	PRO	VIT C	FOL	CA	IR
JAM/JELLY/ PRESERVES							
apple jelly	3½ oz	259	0	–	–	10	–
apricot jam	3½ oz	250	tr	–	–	8	–
blackberry jam	3½ oz	237	1	–	–	–	–
cherry jam	3½ oz	250	tr	1	–	9	–
diet jelly (artificially sweetened)	1 tbsp	6	–	0	tr	1	tr
orange jam	3½ oz	243	tr	4	–	32	–
plum jam	3½ oz	241	tr	–	–	–	–
quince jam	3½ oz	236	tr	–	–	–	–
raspberry jam	3½ oz	248	1	3	–	–	–
raspberry jelly	3½ oz	259	0	–	–	–	–
red currant jelly	3½ oz	265	0	–	–	6	–
red currant jam	3½ oz	237	1	21	–	–	–
rose hip jam	3½ oz	250	tr	51	–	71	–
strawberry jam	3½ oz	234	tr	9	–	10	–
JAVA PLUM							
fresh	1 cup	82	1	19	–	25	tr
JEW'S EAR							
pepeao, dried	½ cup	36	1	tr	–	14	1
pepeao, raw; sliced	1 cup	25	tr	1	–	16	1
JUJUBE							
fresh	3½ oz	105	1	58	–	33	1
KALE							
FRESH chopped, cooked	½ cup	21	1	27	9	47	1
raw; chopped	½ cup	21	1	41	10	46	1
scotch; chopped, cooked	½ cup	18	1	34	9	86	1

FOOD	PORTION	CAL	PRO	VIT C	FOL	CA	IR
FROZEN							
chopped, cooked	½ cup	20	2	16	9	90	1
KEFIR							
kefir	3½ oz	66	3	–	–	–	tr
KIDNEY							
beef; simmered	3 oz	122	22	1	83	15	6
lamb; braised	3 oz	117	20	10	69	15	11
veal; braised	3 oz	139	22	7	18	25	3
KIDNEY BEANS							
CANNED							
kidney beans	1 cup	208	13	3	126	69	3
red	1 cup	216	13	3	129	62	3
DRIED							
california red, raw	1 cup	609	45	8	725	359	17
california red; cooked	1 cup	219	16	2	131	116	5
kidney beans, raw	1 cup	613	43	8	725	263	15
kidney beans; cooked	1 cup	225	15	2	229	0	5
red, raw	1 cup	619	41	8	725	153	12
red; cooked	1 cup	225	15	2	229	50	5
royal red, raw	1 cup	605	47	8	724	241	16
royal red; cooked	1 cup	218	17	2	130	78	5
SPROUTS							
cooked	1 lb	152	22	162	–	84	4
raw	½ cup	27	4	36	–	16	1
KIWI FRUIT							
fresh	1 med	46	1	75	–	20	tr

FOOD	PORTION	CAL	PRO	VIT C	FOL	CA	IR
KOHLRABI							
FRESH							
raw; sliced	½ cup	19	1	43	–	17	tr
sliced, cooked	½ cup	24	1	44	–	20	tr
KUMQUATS							
fresh	1	12	tr	7	–	8	tr
LAMB							
FRESH							
cubed, lean only, raw	1 oz	38	6	–	7	3	1
cubed, lean only; braised	3 oz	190	29	–	18	13	2
cubed, lean only; broiled	3 oz	158	24	–	19	11	2
ground, raw	1 oz	80	5	–	5	4	tr
ground; broiled	3 oz	240	21	–	16	19	2
leg, lean & fat, Choice; roasted	3 oz	219	22	–	17	9	2
loin chop w/ bone lean & fat, Choice, raw	1 chop (3.3 oz)	294	15	–	16	14	2
loin chop w/ bone lean & fat, Choice; broiled	1 chop (2.3 oz)	201	16	–	12	13	1
loin chop w/ bone lean only, Choice; broiled	1 chop (1.6 oz)	100	14	–	11	9	tr
rib chop, lean only, Choice; broiled	3 oz	200	24	–	18	14	2
rib chop, lean & fat, Choice; broiled	3 oz	307	19	–	12	16	2
shank, lean & fat, Choice; braised	3 oz	206	24	–	14	17	2
shank, lean & fat, Choice; roasted	3 oz	191	22	–	19	8	2
shoulder chop w/ bone, lean & fat, Choice, raw	1 chop (4.7 oz)	346	22	–	25	18	2

FOOD	PORTION	CAL	PRO	VIT C	FOL	CA	IR
shoulder chop, w/ bone, lean only, Choice, raw	1 chop (3.5 oz)	133	20	–	24	12	2
shoulder chop, w/ bone, lean only, Choice; braised	1 chop (1.9 oz)	152	19	–	12	14	1
shoulder chop, w/ bone, lean & fat, Choice; braised	1 chop (2.5 oz)	244	21	–	13	18	2
sirloin, lean & fat, Choice; roasted	3 oz	248	21	–	14	10	2
FROZEN							
New Zealand, lean & fat, raw	1 oz	79	5	–	–	4	tr
New Zealand, lean & fat; cooked	3 oz	259	21	–	–	14	2
New Zealand, lean only, raw	1 oz	36	6	–	–	2	tr
New Zealand, lean only; cooked	3 oz	175	25	–	–	11	2

LAMBSQUARTERS

FRESH							
chopped, cooked	½ cup	29	3	33	–	232	1

LEEKS

DRIED							
freeze dried	1 tbsp	1	tr	tr	1	1	tr
FRESH							
chopped, cooked	¼ cup	8	tr	1	6	8	tr
cooked	1 (4.4 oz)	38	1	5	30	37	1
raw	1 (4.4 oz)	76	2	15	80	73	3
raw; chopped	¼ cup	16	tr	3	17	15	1

FOOD	PORTION	CAL	PRO	VIT C	FOL	CA	IR
LEMON							
lemon	1 med	22	1	83	–	66	1
peel	1 tbsp	0	tr	8	–	8	tr
wedge	1	5	tr	21	–	16	tr
JUICE							
bottled	1 tbsp	3	tr	4	2	2	tr
fresh	1 tbsp	4	tr	7	2	1	0
frzn	1 tbsp	3	tr	5	1	1	tr
LENTILS							
DRIED							
cooked	1 cup	231	18	3	358	37	7
raw	1 cup	649	54	12	831	99	17
SPROUTS							
raw	½ cup	40	3	6	38	9	1
LETTUCE							
bibb	1 head (6 oz)	21	2	13	119	–	tr
boston	2 leaves	2	tr	1	11	–	tr
boston	1 head (6 oz)	21	2	13	119	–	tr
iceberg	1 leaf	3	tr	1	11	4	tr
iceberg	1 head (19 oz)	70	5	21	302	102	3
looseleaf; shredded	½ cup	5	tr	5	–	19	tr
romaine; shredded	½ cup	4	tr	7	38	10	tr
LIMA BEANS							
CANNED							
large	1 cup	191	12	0	121	50	4
lima beans	½ cup	93	6	11	–	35	2

FOOD	PORTION	CAL	PRO	VIT C	FOL	CA	IR
DRIED							
baby, raw	1 cup	677	42	0	808	163	13
baby; cooked	1 cup	229	15	0	273	52	4
cooked	½ cup	104	6	9	–	27	2
large, raw	1 cup	602	38	0	703	144	13
large; cooked	1 cup	217	15	0	156	32	5
FROZEN							
cooked	½ cup	94	6	5	–	19	2
fordhook; cooked	½ cup	85	5	11	–	19	1

LIME

FRESH							
lime	1	20	tr	20	6	22	tr
JUICE							
bottled	1 tbsp	3	tr	1	1	2	tr
fresh	1 tbsp	4	tr	5	–	2	0

LINCOD

FRESH							
blue, raw	3½ oz	83	17	–	–	–	–

LING

raw	3 oz	74	16	–	–	29	1

LINGCOD

raw	3 oz	72	15	–	–	12	tr

LIQUOR/LIQUEUR

bloody mary	5 oz	116	1	20	20	10	1
bourbon & soda	4 oz	105	0	0	0	4	–
coffee liqueur	1½ oz	174	0	0	0	1	tr
coffee w/ cream liqueur	1½ oz	154	1	0	0	7	tr
crème de menthe	1½ oz	186	0	–	0	0	tr

FOOD	PORTION	CAL	PRO	VIT C	FOL	CA	IR
daiquiri	2 oz	111	0	1	1	3	tr
gin	1½ oz	110	0	0	0	0	0
gin & tonic	7.5 oz	171	0	1	1	4	–
manhattan	2 oz	128	0	0	tr	1	tr
martini	2½ oz	156	0	0	tr	1	tr
pina colada	4½ oz	262	1	7	14	11	tr
rum	1½ oz	97	0	0	0	0	tr
screwdriver	7 oz	174	1	67	75	16	tr
tequila sunrise	5½ oz	189	1	13	–	10	tr
tom collins	7½ oz	121	tr	4	2	10	–
vodka	1½ oz	97	0	0	0	0	tr
whiskey	1½ oz	105	0	0	0	0	tr
whiskey sour	3 oz	123	tr	11	5	5	tr
whiskey sour mix, not prep	1 pkg (.6 oz)	64	tr	1	0	45	tr
whiskey sour mix; as prep	3.6 oz	169	tr	1	0	47	tr

LIVER

FOOD	PORTION	CAL	PRO	VIT C	FOL	CA	IR
beef; braised	3 oz	137	21	19	184	6	6
beef; pan-fried	3 oz	184	23	19	187	9	5
chicken, raw	1 (1.1 oz)	40	6	11	236	3	3
chicken; stewed	1 cup (5 oz)	219	34	22	1077	20	12
duck, raw	1 (1.5 oz)	60	8	–	24	5	13
goose, raw	1 (3.3 oz)	125	15	–	–	40	–
lamb; braised	3 oz	187	26	3	62	7	7
lamb; fried	3 oz	202	22	11	340	8	9
pork; braised	3 oz	141	22	20	139	9	15
sheep, raw	3½ oz	131	21	31	tr	4	12
turkey, raw	1 (3.6 oz)	140	20	5	752	7	11

FOOD	PORTION	CAL	PRO	VIT C	FOL	CA	IR
turkey; simmered	1 cup (5 oz)	237	34	3	932	15	11
veal; braised	3 oz	140	18	26	645	6	2
veal; fried	3 oz	208	25	18	272	10	4

LOBSTER

FRESH

FOOD	PORTION	CAL	PRO	VIT C	FOL	CA	IR
northern, raw	3 oz	77	77	–	–	–	–
northern, raw	1 lobster (5.3 oz)	136	28	–	–	–	–
northern; cooked	1 cup	142	30	–	16	88	1
northern; cooked	3 oz	83	17	–	9	52	tr
spiny, raw	3 oz	95	18	–	–	41	1
spiny, raw	1 (7.3 oz)	233	43	–	–	102	3

LOGANBERRIES

FOOD	PORTION	CAL	PRO	VIT C	FOL	CA	IR
frzn	1 cup	80	2	23	38	38	1

LOQUATS

FOOD	PORTION	CAL	PRO	VIT C	FOL	CA	IR
fresh	1	5	tr	–	–	2	tr

LONGANS

FOOD	PORTION	CAL	PRO	VIT C	FOL	CA	IR
fresh	1	2	tr	3	–	0	0

LOTUS

FOOD	PORTION	CAL	PRO	VIT C	FOL	CA	IR
root, raw; sliced	10 slices	45	2	36	–	36	1
root; sliced, cooked	10 slices	59	1	24	–	23	1
seeds, dried	1 oz	94	4	0	–	46	1

LUNCHEON MEATS/ COLD CUTS

FOOD	PORTION	CAL	PRO	VIT C	FOL	CA	IR
barbecue loaf, pork & beef	1 oz	49	4	5	–	13	tr

FOOD	PORTION	CAL	PRO	VIT C	FOL	CA	IR
beerwurst, beef	1 slice (1/16" × 2¾")	19	1	1	0	1	tr
beerwurst, beef	1 slice (4" × 1/8")	75	3	3	1	2	tr
beerwurst, pork	1 slice (2¾" × 1/16")	14	1	2	0	0	tr
beerwurst, pork	1 slice (4" × 1/8")	55	4	7	1	2	tr
berliner, pork & beef	1 oz	65	4	2	–	3	tr
blood sausage	1 oz	95	4	–	–	–	–
bologna, beef	1 oz	72	3	4	1	3	tr
bologna, beef & pork	1 oz	89	3	6	1	3	tr
bologna, pork	1 oz	70	4	10	1	3	tr
braunschweiger, pork	1 slice (2½" × ¼")	65	2	2	–	2	2
braunschweiger, pork	1 oz	102	4	3	–	2	3
corned beef loaf	1 oz	46	7	2	–	3	1
dried beef	1 oz	47	–	–	–	2	–
dried beef	5 slices (21 g)	35	–	–	–	1	–
dutch brand loaf, pork & beef	1 oz	68	4	5	–	24	tr
headcheese, pork	1 oz	60	5	6	1	4	tr
honey loaf, pork & beef	1 oz	36	4	6	–	5	tr
honey roll sausage, beef	1 oz	42	4	4	–	2	1
lebanon bologna, beef	1 oz	64	6	10	–	3	
liver cheese, pork	1 oz	86	4	1	–	2	
liverwurst, pork	1 oz	93	4	–	9	7	
luncheon meat, beef	1 oz	87	4	4	–	3	

FOOD	PORTION	CAL	PRO	VIT C	FOL	CA	IR
luncheon meat, pork & beef	1 oz	100	4	4	2	5	tr
luncheon meat, pork, canned	1 oz	95	4	0	2	2	tr
luncheon sausage pork & beef	1 oz	74	4	5	–	3	tr
luxury loaf, pork	1 oz	40	5	6	–	10	tr
mortadella, beef & pork	1 oz	88	5	7	–	5	tr
mother's loaf, pork	1 oz	80	3	0	–	12	tr
new england brand sausage, pork & beef	1 oz	46	5	6	2	2	tr
olive loaf, pork	1 oz	67	3	2	–	31	tr
peppered loaf, pork & beef	1 oz	42	5	7	–	15	tr
pepperoni, pork & beef	1 (9 oz)	1248	53	–	–	25	4
pepperoni, pork & beef	1 slice (.2 oz)	27	1	–	–	1	tr
pickle & pimiento loaf, pork	1 oz	74	3	4	–	27	tr
picnic loaf, pork & beef	1 oz	66	4	5	–	13	tr
salami, cooked, beef & pork	1 oz	71	4	3	1	4	1
salami, hard, pork	1 slice (⅓ oz)	41	2	–	–	1	tr
salami, hard, pork	1 pkg (4 oz)	460	26	–	–	15	1
salami, hard, pork & beef	1 slice (⅓ oz)	42	2	3	–	1	tr
salami, hard, pork & beef	1 pkg (4 oz)	472	26	29	–	8	2
sandwich spread, pork & beef	1 tbsp	35	1	0	–	2	tr
sandwich spread, pork & beef	1 oz	67	2	0	–	3	tr

FOOD	PORTION	CAL	PRO	VIT C	FOL	CA	I
summer sausage, thuringer, cervelat	1 oz	98	5	7	–	2	
TAKE-OUT							
submarine w/ salami, ham, cheese, lettuce, tomato, onion, oil	1	456	22	12	–	189	

LUPINES

DRIED

cooked	1 cup	197	26	–	–	85	
raw	1 cup	668	65	–	–	317	

LYCHEES

fresh	1	6	tr	7	–	0	

MACADAMIA NUTS

dried	1 oz	199	2	–	–	20	
oil roasted	1 oz	204	2	0	–	13	

MACE

ground	1 tsp.	8	tr	–	–	4	

MACKEREL

CANNED

jack	1 can (12.7 oz)	563	84	3	19	870	
jack	1 cup	296	44	2	10	458	
FRESH							
atlantic, raw	3 oz	174	16	tr	–	10	
atlantic; cooked	3 oz	223	20	tr	–	13	
king, raw	3 oz	89	17	–	6	26	
spanish, raw	3 oz	118	16	–	–	10	
spanish; cooked	1 fillet (5.1 oz)	230	34	–	–	19	
spanish; cooked	3 oz	134	20	–	–	11	

FOOD	PORTION	CAL	PRO	VIT C	FOL	CA	IR
MALT							
malt beverage nonalcoholic	12 oz	32	1	–	–	25	tr
MALTED MILK							
POWDER							
chocolate	3 heaping tsp (¾ oz)	83	1	–	4	13	tr
natural flavor	3 heaping tsp (¾ oz)	86	3	0	10	56	tr
PREPARED							
chocolate; as prep w/ whole milk	1 cup	233	9	2	16	304	1
natural flavor: as prep w/ whole milk	1 cup	236	11	2	22	347	tr
MAMMY-APPLE							
fresh	1	431	4	118	–	93	6
MANGO							
fresh	1	135	1	57	–	21	tr
MARGARINE							
REDUCED CALORIE							
diet	1 tsp	17	0	tr	tr	1	–
diet	1 cup	800	1	tr	2	41	–
REGULAR							
corn	1 stick (4 oz)	815	1	tr	1	34	–
corn	1 tsp	34	0	tr	tr	1	–
salted	1 stick (4 oz)	815	1	tr	1	34	tr
salted	1 tsp	39	0	tr	tr	1	0

FOOD	PORTION	CAL	PRO	VIT C	FOL	CA	IR
unsalted	1 stick (4 oz)	809	1	tr	1	20	–
unsalted	1 tsp	34	0	tr	tr	1	–
SOFT corn	1 tsp	34	0	tr	tr	1	–
corn	1 cup	1626	2	tr	2	60	–
safflower	1 tsp	34	0	tr	tr	1	
safflower	1 cup	1626	2	tr	2	60	–
soybean, unsalted	1 cup	1626	2	tr	2	60	–
soybean, unsalted	1 tsp	34	0	tr	tr	1	–
soybean, salted	1 tsp	34	0	tr	tr	1	–
soybean, salted	1 cup	1626	2	tr	2	60	–
tub, salted	1 cup	1626	2	tr	2	60	–
tub, salted	1 tsp	34	0	tr	tr	1	–
tub, unsalted	1 cup	1626	0	tr	2	60	–
tub, unsalted	1 tsp	34	0	tr	tr	1	–
SQUEEZE soybean & cottonseed	1 tsp	34	tr	tr	tr	3	–

MARJORAM

FOOD	PORTION	CAL	PRO	VIT C	FOL	CA	IR
dried	1 tsp	2	tr	–	–	12	1

MAYONNAISE

FOOD	PORTION	CAL	PRO	VIT C	FOL	CA	IR
REDUCED CALORIE reduced calorie	1 tbsp	34	0	–	–	–	–
reduced calorie	1 cup	556	1	–	–	–	–
REGULAR mayonnaise	1 tbsp	99	tr	–	–	2	t
mayonnaise	1 cup	1577	2	–	–	40	1
sandwich spread	1 tbsp	60	tr	–	–	–	–

FOOD	PORTION	CAL	PRO	VIT C	FOL	CA	IR
MAYONNAISE TYPE SALAD DRESSING							
REDUCED CALORIE							
reduced calorie w/o cholesterol	1 cup	1084	tr	–	–	–	–
reduced calorie w/o cholesterol	1 tbsp	68	7	–	–	–	–
REGULAR							
home recipe	1 tbsp	25	1	tr	–	13	tr
home recipe	1 cup	400	11	2	–	214	1
mayonnaise type salad dressing	1 cup	916	2	–	–	33	1
mayonnaise type salad dressing	1 tbsp	57	tr	–	–	–	–
MEAT SUBSTITUTES							
simulated sausage	1 link (25 g)	64	5	0	7	16	1
simulated sausage	1 patty (38 g)	97	7	0	10	24	1
MELON							
FROZEN							
melon balls	1 cup	55	1	11	45	17	1
MEXICAN FOOD							
CANNED							
refried beans	½ cup	134	8	8	–	59	2
READY-TO-USE							
tortilla, corn	1 (1 oz)	65	2	0	–	42	1
TAKE-OUT							
burrito w/ apple	1 sm (2.6 oz)	231	3	tr	4	15	1
burrito w/ apple	1 lg (5.4 oz)	484	5	2	4	32	2

FOOD	PORTION	CAL	PRO	VIT C	FOL	CA	IR
burrito w/ cherry	1 sm (2.6 oz)	231	3	tr	4	15	1
burrito w/ cherry	1 lg (5.4 oz)	484	5	2	4	32	2
burrito w/ beans	2 (7.6 oz)	448	14	2	118	113	5
burrito w/ beans & cheese	2 (6.5 oz)	377	15	2	81	214	2
burrito w/ beans & chili peppers	2 (7.2 oz)	413	16	1	118	100	5
burrito w/ beans & meat	2 (8.1 oz)	508	22	2	73	105	5
burrito w/ beef	2 (7.7 oz)	523	27	1	39	84	6
burrito w/ beef & chili peppers	2 (7.1 oz)	426	22	2	37	87	4
burrito w/ beef, cheese & chili peppers	2 (10.7 oz)	634	41	4	58	223	8
burrito w/ beans, cheese & beef	2 (7.1 oz)	331	15	5	61	131	4
burrito w/ beans, cheese & chili peppers	2 (11.8 oz)	663	33	7	146	288	8
chimichanga w/ beef	1 (6.1 oz)	425	20	5	31	63	5
chimichanga w/ beef & cheese	1 (6.4 oz)	443	20	3	34	238	4
chimichanga w/ beef & red chili peppers	1 (6.7 oz)	424	18	tr	34	71	4
chimichanga w/ beef, cheese & red chili peppers	1 (6.3 oz)	364	15	2	33	218	3
enchilada w/ cheese	1 (5.7 oz)	320	10	tr	34	324	1
enchilada w/ cheese & beef	1 (6.7 oz)	324	12	1	192	228	3
enchirito w/ cheese, beef & beans	1 (6.8 oz)	344	18	5	254	217	2
frijoles w/ cheese	1 cup (5.9 oz)	226	11	2	111	188	2

FOOD	PORTION	CAL	PRO	VIT C	FOL	CA	IR
nachos w/ cheese	6 to 8 (4 oz)	345	9	1	10	272	1
nachos w/ cheese & jalapeno peppers	6 to 8 (7.2 oz)	607	17	tr	19	620	2
nachos w/ cheese, beans, ground beef & peppers	6 to 8 (8.9 oz)	568	20	5	39	384	3
nachos w/ cinnamon & sugar	6 to 8 (3.8 oz)	592	7	8	7	85	3
taco	1 sm (6 oz)	370	21	2	23	221	2
taco salad	1½ cups	279	13	4	40	192	2
taco salad w/ chili con carne	1½ cups	288	17	3	64	246	3
tostada w/ beans & cheese	1 (5.1 oz)	223	10	1	75	211	2
tostada w/ beans, beef & cheese	1 (7.9 oz)	334	16	4	97	190	2
tostada w/ beef & cheese	1 (5.7 oz)	315	19	3	15	217	3
tostada w/ guacamole	2 (9.2 oz)	360	12	4	110	424	2

MILK

CANNED
condensed, sweetened	1 oz	123	3	1	4	108	tr
condensed, sweetened	1 cup	982	24	8	34	868	1
evaporated	½ cup	169	9	2	10	329	tr
evaporated, skim	½ cup	99	10	2	11	369	tr

DRIED
buttermilk	1 tbsp	25	2	tr	3	77	tr
nonfat, instantized	1 pkg (3.2 oz)	244	32	5	45	837	tr

LIQUID, LOWFAT
1% protein fortified	1 cup	119	10	3	15	349	tr
1%	1 cup	102	8	2	12	300	tr

FOOD	PORTION	CAL	PRO	VIT C	FOL	CA	IR
1%	1 qt	409	32	9	50	1200	tr
1%, protein fortified	1 qt	477	39	11	58	1397	1
2%	1 cup	121	8	2	12	297	tr
2%	1 qt	485	33	9	50	1187	tr
buttermilk	1 cup	99	8	2	–	285	tr
buttermilk	1 qt	396	32	10	–	1141	tr
LIQUID, REGULAR							
buffalo	3½ oz	112	4	3	–	195	tr
camel milk	3½ oz	80	5	–	–	132	–
donkey milk	3½ oz	43	2	2	–	110	tr
goat	1 cup	168	9	3	1	326	tr
goat	1 qt	672	35	13	6	1303	tr
human	1 cup	171	3	12	13	79	tr
indian buffalo	1 cup	236	9	5	14	412	tr
low sodium	1 cup	149	8	–	–	246	–
mare milk	3½ oz	49	2	15	–	110	tr
sheep	1 cup	264	15	10	–	474	tr
whole	1 cup	150	8	2	12	291	tr
LIQUID, SKIM							
skim	1 cup	86	8	2	13	302	tr
skim	1 qt	342	33	10	51	1209	1
skim, protein fortified	1 cup	100	10	3	15	352	tr
skim, protein fortified	1 qt	400	39	11	59	1407	1

MILK DRINKS

FOOD	PORTION	CAL	PRO	VIT C	FOL	CA	IR
chocolate milk	1 cup	208	8	2	12	280	1
chocolate milk	1 qt	833	32	9	47	1121	2
chocolate milk 1% fat	1 cup	158	8	2	12	287	1
chocolate milk, 1% fat	1 qt	630	32	9	48	1147	2
chocolate milk, 2% fat	1 cup	179	8	2	12	284	1

FOOD	PORTION	CAL	PRO	VIT C	FOL	CA	IR
strawberry flavor mix; as prep w/ whole milk	9 oz	234	8	2	12	292	tr

MILK SUBSTITUTES

FOOD	PORTION	CAL	PRO	VIT C	FOL	CA	IR
imitation milk	1 cup	150	4	0	0	79	1
imitation milk	1 qt	600	17	0	0	317	4

MILKFISH

FRESH

FOOD	PORTION	CAL	PRO	VIT C	FOL	CA	IR
raw	3 oz	126	17	–	–	43	tr

MILK SHAKE

FOOD	PORTION	CAL	PRO	VIT C	FOL	CA	IR
chocolate	10 oz	360	10	1	10	319	1
chocolate thick shake	10.6 oz	356	9	0	15	396	1
strawberry	10 oz	319	10	2	9	320	tr
vanilla	10 oz	314	10	2	9	344	tr
vanilla thick shake	11 oz	350	12	0	21	457	tr

MILLET

FOOD	PORTION	CAL	PRO	VIT C	FOL	CA	IR
cooked	½ cup	143	4	0	–	4	tr
raw	½ cup	378	11	0	–	8	3

MISO

FOOD	PORTION	CAL	PRO	VIT C	FOL	CA	IR
miso	½ cup	284	16	0	46	92	4

MOLASSES

FOOD	PORTION	CAL	PRO	VIT C	FOL	CA	IR
blackstrap	2 tbsp	85	0	0	–	274	10
molasses	2 tbsp	85	0	0	–	274	10

MONKFISH

FRESH

FOOD	PORTION	CAL	PRO	VIT C	FOL	CA	IR
raw	3 oz	64	12	–	–	7	tr

FOOD	PORTION	CAL	PRO	VIT C	FOL	CA	IR
MOOSE							
raw	1 oz	29	6	1	–	1	1
roasted	3 oz	114	25	4	–	5	4
MOTH BEANS							
DRIED							
cooked	1 cup	207	14	2	–	6	6
raw	1 cup	673	45	8	–	294	21
MUFFIN							
HOME RECIPE							
blueberry	1 (1.5 oz)	135	3	1	–	54	1
bran	1 (1.5 oz)	125	3	3	–	60	1
MIX							
blueberry	1 (1.5 oz)	140	3	tr	–	15	1
bran	1 (1.5 oz)	140	3	0	–	27	2
corn	1 (1.5 oz)	145	3	tr	–	30	1
MULBERRIES							
fresh	1 cup	61	2	51	–	55	3
MULLET							
FRESH							
striped, raw	3 oz	99	16	–	7	34	1
striped; cooked	3 oz	127	21	–	–	26	1
MUNG BEANS							
DRIED							
cooked	1 cup	213	14	2	321	55	3
raw	1 cup	719	49	10	1294	273	14
SPROUTS							
canned	½ cup	8	1	tr	6	9	tr
cooked	½ cup	13	1	7	–	7	tr
raw	½ cup	16	2	7	32	7	tr

FOOD	PORTION	CAL	PRO	VIT C	FOL	CA	IR
stir fried	½ cup	31	3	–	–	8	1

MUNGO BEANS

DRIED
cooked	1 cup	190	14	2	170	95	3
raw	1 cup	726	52	10	1301	406	14

MUSHROOMS

CANNED
chanterelle	3½ oz	12	1	3	–	5	1
pieces	½ cup	19	1	–	10	–	1
whole	1 (.4 oz)	3	tr	–	2	–	tr

DRIED
chanterelle	3½ oz	89	17	2	–	85	17
shitake	4 (½ oz)	44	1	–	–	2	tr

FRESH
chanterelle	3½ oz	11	2	6	–	8	7
morel	3½ oz	9	2	5	–	11	1
raw	1 (½ oz)	5	tr	1	4	1	tr
raw; sliced	½ cup	9	1	1	7	2	tr
shitake; cooked	4 (2.5 oz)	40	1	tr	–	2	tr
sliced, cooked	½ cup	21	2	3	14	4	1
whole; cooked	1 (.4 oz)	3	tr	1	2	1	tr

MUSKRAT

raw	1 oz	46	6	1	–	7	–
roasted	3 oz	156	20	5	–	24	–

MUSSELS

FRESH
blue, raw	3 oz	73	10	–	–	22	3
blue, raw	1 cup	129	18	–	–	39	6
blue; cooked	3 oz	147	20	–	–	28	6

FOOD	PORTION	CAL	PRO	VIT C	FOL	CA	IR
MUSTARD							
yellow	1 tsp	5	tr	0	–	4	tr
DRY mustard seed, yellow	1 tsp	15	1	–	–	17	tr
MUSTARD GREENS							
FRESH chopped, cooked	½ cup	11	2	18	–	52	tr
raw; chopped	½ cup	7	1	20	–	29	tr
FROZEN chopped; cooked	½ cup	14	2	10	–	75	1
NATTO							
natto	½ cup	187	16	11	–	191	8
NAVY BEANS							
CANNED navy	1 cup	296	20	2	163	123	5
DRIED cooked	1 cup	259	16	2	255	128	5
raw	1 cup	697	46	6	769	322	13
SPROUTS cooked	3½ oz	78	–	–	–	16	–
raw	½ cup	35	–	–	–	8	–
NECTARINE							
fresh	1	67	1	7	5	6	tr
NOODLES							
DRY cellophane	1 cup	492	tr	0	–	35	3
chow mein	1 cup	237	4	0	10	9	2
egg	½ cup	145	5	0	11	12	2
egg; cooked	1 cup	212	8	0	11	19	3

FOOD	PORTION	CAL	PRO	VIT C	FOL	CA	IR
japanese soba	2 oz	192	8	0	34	20	2
japanese soba; cooked	½ cup	56	3	0	4	2	tr
japanese somen	2 oz.	203	6	0	8	13	tr
japanese somen; cooked	½ cup	115	4	0	1	7	tr
spinach/egg	1 cup	145	6	0	34	21	2
spinach/egg; cooked	1 cup	211	8	0	34	30	2

NUTMEG
| ground | 1 tsp | 12 | tr | – | – | 4 | tr |

NUTS MIXED
dry roasted w/ peanuts, salted	1 oz	169	5	tr	14	20	1
dry roasted w/ peanuts	1 oz	169	5	tr	14	20	1
oil roasted w/ peanuts	1 oz	175	5	tr	24	31	1
oil roasted, w/o peanuts	1 oz	175	4	tr	16	30	1
oil roasted w/ peanuts, salted	1 oz	175	5	tr	24	31	1
oil roasted w/o peanuts, salted	1 oz	175	4	tr	0	30	1

OCTOPUS
FRESH
| raw | 3 oz | 70 | 13 | – | – | 45 | 5 |

OHELOBERRIES
| fresh | 1 cup | 39 | 1 | 8 | – | 10 | tr |

OIL
almond	1 cup	1927	0	–	–	–	–
almond	1 tbsp	120	0	–	–	–	–
apricot kernel	1 cup	1927	0	–	–	–	–
apricot kernel	1 tbsp	120	0	–	–	–	–

FOOD	PORTION	CAL	PRO	VIT C	FOL	CA	IR
canola	1 tbsp	120	0	–	–	–	–
canola	1 cup	1927	0	–	–	–	–
coconut	1 tbsp	120	0	–	–	tr	–
corn	1 cup	1927	0	–	–	–	–
corn	1 tbsp	120	0	–	–	–	–
cottonseed	1 cup	1927	0	–	–	–	–
cottonseed	1 tbsp	120	0	–	–	–	–
cupu assu	1 tbsp	120	0	–	–	–	–
grapeseed	1 tbsp	120	0	–	–	–	–
hazelnut	1 cup	1927	0	–	–	–	–
hazelnut	1 tbsp	120	0	–	–	–	–
herring	3½ oz	945	0	–	–	–	–
olive	1 tbsp	119	0	–	–	tr	tr
olive	1 cup	1909	0	–	–	tr	1
palm	1 cup	1927	0	–	–	–	tr
palm	1 tbsp	120	0	–	–	–	0
palm kernel	1 tbsp	120	0	–	–	–	–
palm kernel	1 cup	1927	0	–	–	–	–
palm, babassu	1 tbsp	120	0	–	–	–	–
peanut	1 cup	1909	0	–	–	tr	tr
peanut	1 tbsp	119	0	–	–	tr	0
poppyseed	1 tbsp	120	0	–	–	–	–
pumpkin seed	3½ oz	925	0	–	–	–	–
rice bran	1 tbsp	120	0	–	–	–	tr
safflower	1 tbsp	120	0	–	–	–	–
safflower	1 cup	1927	0	–	–	–	–
sesame	1 tbsp	120	0	–	–	–	–
shark	3½ oz	945	0	–	–	–	–
sheanut	1 tbsp	120	0	–	–	–	–

FOOD	PORTION	CAL	PRO	VIT C	FOL	CA	IR
soybean	1 tbsp	120	0	–	–	tr	0
soybean	1 cup	1927	0	–	–	tr	tr
sunflower	1 tbsp	120	0	–	–	–	–
sunflower	1 cup	1927	0	–	–	–	–
teaseed	1 tbsp	120	0	–	–	–	–
tomatoseed	1 tbsp	120	0	–	–	–	–
vegetable, soybean & cottonseed	1 tbsp	120	0	–	–	–	–
vegetable, soybean & cottonseed	1 cup	1927	0	–	–	–	–
walnut	1 cup	1927	0	–	–	–	–
walnut	1 tbsp	120	0	–	–	–	–
whale	3½ oz	945	0	–	–	–	–
wheat germ	1 tbsp	120	0	–	–	–	–

OKRA

FRESH

FOOD	PORTION	CAL	PRO	VIT C	FOL	CA	IR
raw	8 pods	36	2	20	83	77	1
raw; sliced	½ cup	19	1	11	44	41	tr
sliced, cooked	½ cup	25	1	13	37	50	tr
sliced, cooked	8 pods	27	2	14	39	54	tr

FROZEN

FOOD	PORTION	CAL	PRO	VIT C	FOL	CA	IR
sliced; cooked	½ cup	34	2	11	134	88	1
sliced; cooked	1 pkg (10 oz)	94	5	31	371	245	2

OLIVES

FOOD	PORTION	CAL	PRO	VIT C	FOL	CA	IR
green	4 med	15	tr	0	–	8	tr
green	3 extra lg	15	tr	0	–	8	tr
ripe	1 sm	4	tr	0	0	3	tr
ripe	1 lg	5	tr	0	0	4	tr

FOOD	PORTION	CAL	PRO	VIT C	FOL	CA	IR
ONION							
CANNED							
chopped	½ cup	21	1	–	–	51	tr
whole	1 (2.2 oz)	12	1	–	–	29	tr
DRIED							
flakes	1 tbsp	16	tr	4	8	13	tr
powder	1 tsp	7	tr	0	–	8	tr
FRESH							
chopped, cooked	½ cup	29	1	6	16	29	tr
raw; chopped	1 tbsp	3	tr	1	2	2	tr
raw; chopped	½ cup	27	1	7	15	20	tr
scallions, raw; chopped	1 tbsp	2	tr	3	4	4	tr
scallions, raw; sliced	½ cup	13	1	23	32	30	1
welsh, raw	3½ oz	34	2	27	–	18	–
FROZEN							
chopped; cooked	1 tbsp	4	tr	tr	0	2	tr
chopped; cooked	½ cup	30	tr	3	14	17	tr
rings	7 (2.5 oz)	285	4	1	9	21	1
rings; cooked	2 (.7 oz)	81	1	tr	3	6	tr
whole; cooked	3½ oz	28	tr	5	13	27	tr
TAKE-OUT							
rings; breaded & fried	8 to 9	275	4	tr	11	73	tr
OPOSSUM							
roasted	3 oz	188	26	–	–	–	–
ORANGE							
FRESH							
california valencia	1	59	1	59	47	48	tr
california navel	1	65	1	80	47	56	tr
florida	1	69	1	68	26	65	tr
peel	1 tbsp	6	tr	8	–	10	tr

FOOD	PORTION	CAL	PRO	VIT C	FOL	CA	IR
sections	1 cup	85	2	96	55	52	tr
JUICE							
canned	1 cup	104	1	86	–	21	1
chilled	1 cup	110	2	82	45	24	tr
fresh	1 cup	111	2	124	–	27	1
frzn, not prep	6 oz	339	5	294	331	67	1
frzn; as prep	1 cup	112	2	97	109	22	tr
mandarin orange	3½ oz	47	1	32	–	19	tr
orange drink	6 oz	94	0	64	–	12	1

OREGANO

FOOD	PORTION	CAL	PRO	VIT C	FOL	CA	IR
ground	1 tsp	5	tr	–	–	24	1

ORIENTAL FOOD

FOOD	PORTION	CAL	PRO	VIT C	FOL	CA	IR
CANNED							
chow mein chicken	1 cup	95	7	tr	–	45	1
HOME RECIPE							
chop suey w/ beef & pork	1 cup	300	26	33	–	81	5
chow mein chicken	1 cup	255	31	10	–	58	3

OYSTERS

FOOD	PORTION	CAL	PRO	VIT C	FOL	CA	IR
CANNED							
eastern	1 cup	170	18	–	22	111	17
eastern	3 oz	58	6	–	8	38	6
FRESH							
eastern, raw	6 med	58	6	–	8	38	6
eastern, raw	1 cup	170	18	–	25	111	17
eastern; cooked	6 med	58	6	–	8	38	6
eastern; cooked	3 oz	117	12	–	15	76	11
pacific, raw	3 oz	69	8	–	–	7	4
pacific, raw	1 med	41	5	–	–	4	3

FOOD	PORTION	CAL	PRO	VIT C	FOL	CA	IR
HOME RECIPE							
eastern; breaded & fried	3 oz	167	7	–	12	53	6
eastern; breaded & fried	6 medium	173	8	–	12	54	6
TAKE-OUT							
battered & fried	6 (4.9 oz)	368	13	4	13	27	4
breaded & fried	6 (4.9 oz)	368	13	4	13	27	4

PANCAKE/WAFFLE SYRUP

FOOD	PORTION	CAL	PRO	VIT C	FOL	CA	IR
low calorie	1 tbsp	12	0	0	0	–	–
maple	2 tbsp	122	0	0	–	1	tr

PANCAKES

FOOD	PORTION	CAL	PRO	VIT C	FOL	CA	IR
HOME RECIPE							
plain	1 (4" diam)	60	2	tr	–	5	1
MIX							
buckwheat	1 (4" diam)	55	2	tr	–	59	tr
TAKE-OUT							
w/ butter & syrup	3	519	8	3	34	128	3

PAPAYA

FOOD	PORTION	CAL	PRO	VIT C	FOL	CA	IR
FRESH							
cubed	1 cup	54	1	87	–	33	tr
papaya	1	117	2	188	–	72	tr
JUICE							
nectar	1 cup	142	tr	8	5	24	1

PAPRIKA

FOOD	PORTION	CAL	PRO	VIT C	FOL	CA	IR
paprika	1 tsp	6	tr	1	–	4	1

PARSLEY

FOOD	PORTION	CAL	PRO	VIT C	FOL	CA	IR
dried	1 tsp	1	tr	tr	–	4	tr
dried	1 tbsp	1	tr	1	6	1	tr
fresh, raw; chopped	½ cup	11	1	40	46	41	2

FOOD	PORTION	CAL	PRO	VIT C	FOL	CA	IR
PARSNIPS							
FRESH							
cooked	1 (5.6 oz)	130	2	21	93	59	1
cooked, sliced	½ cup	63	1	10	45	29	tr
raw; sliced	½ cup	50	1	11	45	24	tr
PASSION FRUIT							
purple	1	18	tr	5	–	2	tr
JUICE							
purple	1 cup	126	1	74	–	9	1
yellow	1 cup	149	2	45	–	9	1
PASTA							
DRY							
corn	2 oz	204	4	0	26	4	tr
corn; cooked	1 cup	176	4	0	9	2	tr
elbows	1 cup	389	13	0	19	19	4
elbows; cooked	1 cup	197	7	0	10	10	2
protein-fortified	1 cup	348	18	0	18	36	4
protein-fortified; cooked	1 cup	188	9	0	12	12	tr
shells	1 cup	389	13	0	19	19	4
shells; cooked	1 cup	197	7	0	10	10	2
spaghetti	2 oz	211	7	0	10	10	2
spaghetti, protein fortified	2 oz	214	11	0	11	22	2
spaghetti, protein fortified; cooked	1 cup	229	11	0	15	14	1
spaghetti; cooked	1 cup	197	7	0	10	10	2
spinach spaghetti	2 oz	212	8	0	27	33	1
spinach spaghetti; cooked	1 cup	183	6	0	16	42	1
spirals	1 cup	389	13	0	19	19	4
spirals; cooked	1 cup	197	7	0	10	10	2

FOOD	PORTION	CAL	PRO	VIT C	FOL	CA	IR
vegetable	1 cup	308	11	0	14	29	4
vegetable; cooked	1 cup	171	6	0	7	15	tr
whole wheat	1 cup	365	15	0	60	42	4
whole wheat spaghetti	2 oz	198	8	0	32	23	2
whole wheat spaghetti; cooked	1 cup	174	7	0	7	21	1
whole wheat; cooked	1 cup	174	7	0	7	21	1
FRESH plain made w/ egg	4.5 oz	368	14	0	–	19	4
plain made w/ egg; cooked	2 oz	75	3	0	–	4	tr
spinach made w/ egg	4.5 oz	370	14	0	–	55	4
spinach made w/ egg; cooked	2 oz	74	3	0	–	10	tr
HOME RECIPE made w/ egg; cooked	2 oz	74	3	0	11	6	tr

PASTA DINNERS

FOOD	PORTION	CAL	PRO	VIT C	FOL	CA	IR
CANNED macaroni & cheese	1 cup	230	9	tr	–	199	1
HOME RECIPE macaroni & cheese	1 cup	430	17	1	–	362	2
spaghetti w/ meatballs & tomato sauce	1 cup	330	19	22	–	124	4

PATE

FOOD	PORTION	CAL	PRO	VIT C	FOL	CA	IR
CANNED chicken liver	1 tbsp	109	2	–	–	1	1
chicken liver	1 oz	238	4	–	–	3	3
goose liver, smoked	1 tbsp	60	1	–	–	–	–
goose liver, smoked	1 oz	131	3	–	–	–	–
liver	1 tbsp	41	5	0	8	9	1
liver	1 oz	90	4	0	17	20	2

FOOD	PORTION	CAL	PRO	VIT C	FOL	CA	IR
PEACH							
halves in heavy syrup	1 half	60	tr	2	3	8	tr
halves in light syrup	1 half	44	tr	2	3	3	tr
halves juice pack	1 half	34	tr	3	–	15	tr
halves water pack	1 half	18	tr	2	3	2	tr
spiced in heavy syrup	1 fruit	66	tr	5	–	5	tr
spiced in heavy syrup	1 cup	180	1	13	–	15	1
DRIED							
halves	10	311	5	6	–	37	5
halves	1 cup	383	6	8	–	45	7
halves; cooked w/ sugar	½ cup	139	1	5	tr	11	2
halves; cooked w/o sugar	½ cup	99	1	5	tr	12	2
FRESH							
peach	1	37	1	6	3	5	tr
sliced	1 cup	73	1	11	6	9	tr
FROZEN							
slices, sweetened	1 cup	235	2	235	–	6	1
JUICE							
nectar	1 cup	134	1	13	–	13	tr
PEANUT BUTTER							
chunk style	1 cup	1520	62	0	237	105	5
chunk style	2 tbsp	188	8	0	29	13	1
smooth	1 tbsp	95	5	0	13	5	tr
smooth	1 cup	1526	73	0	212	85	5
smooth w/o salt	1 tbsp	95	5	0	13	5	tr
smooth w/o salt	1 cup	1526	73	0	212	85	5
PEANUTS							
boiled	½ cup	102	4	0	24	18	tr
dried	1 oz	161	7	0	29	17	1

FOOD	PORTION	CAL	PRO	VIT C	FOL	CA	IF
dry roasted	1 cup	855	35	0	212	79	
dry roasted	1 oz	164	7	0	41	15	
oil roasted	1 oz	165	8	0	30	24	
oil roasted	1 oz	165	14	0	30	24	
oil roasted	1 cup	841	39	0	153	125	
spanish, oil roasted	1 oz	162	8	0	35	28	
spanish, oil roasted	1 cup	851	41	0	185	147	
valencia, oil roasted	1 cup	848	39	0	181	78	
valencia, oil roasted	1 oz	165	8	0	35	15	
virginia, oil roasted	1 oz	161	8	0	35	24	
virginia, oil roasted	1 cup	826	37	0	179	123	

PEAR

CANNED
halves in heavy syrup	1 cup	188	1	3	3	12	
halves in heavy syrup	1 half	68	tr	1	1	4	
halves in light syrup	1 half	45	tr	1	1	4	
halves juice pack	1 cup	123	1	4	–	21	
halves water pack	1 half	22	tr	1	1	–	

DRIED
halves	10	459	3	12	–	59	
halves	1 cup	472	3	13	–	60	
halves; cooked w/ sugar	½ cup	196	1	5	0	22	
halves; cooked w/o sugar	½ cup	163	tr	5	0	21	

FRESH
pear	1	98	1	7	12	19	

JUICE
nectar	1 cup	149	tr	3	–	11	

PEAS

CANNED
green	½ cup	59	4	8	38	17	

FOOD	PORTION	CAL	PRO	VIT C	FOL	CA	IR
DRIED							
split, raw	1 cup	671	48	4	539	108	9
split; cooked	1 cup	231	16	1	127	26	3
FRESH							
edible-pod, raw	½ cup	30	2	43	–	36	2
edible-pod; cooked	½ cup	34	3	38	–	33	2
green, raw	½ cup	63	4	31	47	19	1
green; cooked	½ cup	67	4	11	51	22	1
FROZEN							
edible-pod; cooked	1 pkg (10 oz)	132	9	56	–	150	6
edible-pod; cooked	½ cup	42	3	18	–	48	2
green; cooked	½ cup	63	4	8	47	19	1
SPROUTS							
raw	½ cup	77	5	6	87	21	1
PECANS							
dried	1 oz	190	19	1	11	10	1
dry roasted	1 oz	187	2	–	12	10	1
dry roasted, salted	1 oz	187	2	–	12	10	1
halves, dried	1 cup	721	8	2	42	39	2
oil roasted	1 oz	195	2	–	–	10	1
oil roasted, salted	1 oz	195	2	–	–	10	1
PEPPER							
black	1 tsp	5	tr	–	–	9	1
cayenne	1 tsp	6	tr	1	–	3	tr
red	1 tsp	6	tr	1	–	3	tr
white	1 tsp	7	tr	–	–	6	tr
PEPPERS							
CANNED							
chili, green, hot	1 (2.6 oz)	18	1	50	–	5	tr

FOOD	PORTION	CAL	PRO	VIT C	FOL	CA	IR
chili, green, hot, raw	1	18	1	109	11	8	1
chili, green, hot; chopped	½ cup	17	1	46	–	5	tr
chili, red, hot	1 (2.6 oz)	18	1	50	–	5	tr
chili, red, hot; chopped	½ cup	17	1	46	–	5	tr
green, halves	½ cup	13	1	33	–	28	1
jalapeno; chopped	½ cup	17	1	9	–	18	2
red, halves	½ cup	13	1	33	–	28	1
DRIED							
green	1 tbsp	1	tr	8	1	1	tr
red	1 tbsp	1	tr	8	1	1	tr
FRESH							
chili, green, hot, raw; chopped	½ cup	30	2	182	18	13	1
chili, red, hot, raw	1 (1.6 oz)	18	1	109	11	8	1
chili, red, raw; chopped	½ cup	30	2	182	18	13	1
green, raw	1 (2.6)	18	1	95	13	4	1
green; cooked	1 (2.6 oz)	13	tr	81	7	3	1
green; cooked	½ cup	13	tr	76	7	3	1
red, raw	1 (2.6 oz)	18	1	95	16	4	1
red; chopped, cooked	½ cup	12	tr	64	11	3	1
red; cooked	1 (2.6 oz)	13	tr	81	7	3	1
FROZEN							
green, chopped; not prep	1 oz	6	tr	16	4	3	tr
red, chopped; not prep	1 oz	6	tr	16	4	3	tr

PERCH

FOOD	PORTION	CAL	PRO	VIT C	FOL	CA	IR
FRESH							
cooked	1 fillet (1.6 oz)	54	11	–	–	47	1
cooked	3 oz	99	21	–	–	87	1
ocean perch, Atlantic, raw	3 oz	80	16	–	–	91	1

FOOD	PORTION	CAL	PRO	VIT C	FOL	CA	IR
ocean perch, Atlantic; cooked	1 fillet (1.8 oz)	60	12	–	–	69	1
ocean perch, Atlantic; cooked	3 oz	103	20	–	–	117	1
raw	3 oz	77	16	–	–	68	1
red, raw	3½ oz	114	18	1	–	22	1

PERSIMMONS

dried, japanese	1	93	tr	0	–	8	tr
fresh	1	32	tr	17	–	7	1
fresh, japanese	1	118	1	13	13	13	tr

PHEASANT

FRESH

breast w/o skin, raw	½ breast (6.4 oz)	243	44	11	–	6	1
leg w/o skin, raw	1 (3.6 oz)	143	24	–	–	31	2
w/ skin, raw	½ pheasant (14 oz)	723	91	21	–	50	5
w/o skin, raw	½ pheasant (12.4 oz)	470	83	21	–	45	4

PICKLES

dill	1 (2.3 oz)	5	tr	4	1	17	1
gherkins	3½ oz	21	1	2	–	30	2
quick sour; sliced	½ oz	10	tr	1	–	3	tr
sweet gherkin	1 sm (½ oz)	20	tr	1	–	2	tr

PIE

CANNED FILLING

pumpkin pie mix	1 cup	282	1	5	–	49	1

FOOD	PORTION	CAL	PRO	VIT C	FOL	CA	IR
HOME RECIPE							
pecan	⅙ of 9" pie	575	7	0	–	65	5
READY-TO-USE							
apple	⅙ of 9" pie	405	3	2	–	13	2
blueberry	⅙ of 9" pie	380	4	6	–	17	2
cherry	⅙ of 9" pie	410	4	0	–	22	2
creme	⅙ of 9" pie	455	3	0	–	46	1
custard	⅙ of 9" pie	330	9	0	–	146	2
lemon meringue	⅙ of 9" pie	355	5	4	–	20	1
peach	⅙ of 9" pie	405	4	5	–	167	2
pumpkin	⅙ of 9" pie	320	6	0	–	78	1
SNACK							
apple	1 (3 oz)	266	2	1	4	127	tr
cherry	1 (3 oz)	266	2	1	4	127	tr
lemon	1 (3 oz)	266	2	1	4	127	tr

PIE CRUST

FOOD	PORTION	CAL	PRO	VIT C	FOL	CA	IR
HOME RECIPE							
9-inch crust	1	900	11	0	–	25	5
MIX							
as prep	2 crusts	1485	20	0	–	131	9

PIG'S EARS AND FEET

FOOD	PORTION	CAL	PRO	VIT C	FOL	CA	IR
ears, frzn, raw	1 ear (4 oz)	263	–	–	–	23	–

FOOD	PORTION	CAL	PRO	VIT C	FOL	CA	IR
ears, frzn; simmered	1 ear (3.7 oz)	183	18	0	–	20	2
feet, pickled	1 oz	58	4	0	–	9	–
feet, pickled	1 lb	923	61	0	–	145	–
feet; simmered	2.5 oz	138	14	0	–	32	–

PIGEON PEAS

DRIED

FOOD	PORTION	CAL	PRO	VIT C	FOL	CA	IR
cooked	½ cup	86	5	22	–	27	1
cooked	1 cup	204	11	0	186	72	2
raw	1 cup	704	44	0	935	267	11

PIKE

FRESH

FOOD	PORTION	CAL	PRO	VIT C	FOL	CA	IR
northern, raw	3 oz	75	16	3	–	48	tr
northern; cooked	½ fillet (5.4 oz)	176	38	6	–	113	1
northern; cooked	3 oz	96	21	–	3	62	1
walleye red, raw	3 oz	79	16	–	–	94	1

PILLNUTS

FOOD	PORTION	CAL	PRO	VIT C	FOL	CA	IR
pillnuts-canarytree, dried	1 oz	204	3	–	–	41	1

PINE NUTS

FOOD	PORTION	CAL	PRO	VIT C	FOL	CA	IR
pignolia, dried	1 oz	146	7	–	–	7	3
pignolia, dried	1 tbsp	51	2	–	–	3	1
pinyon, dried	1 oz	161	3	1	–	2	1

PINEAPPLE

CANNED

FOOD	PORTION	CAL	PRO	VIT C	FOL	CA	IR
chunks in heavy syrup	1 cup	199	1	19	12	35	1
chunks juice pack	1 cup	150	1	24	–	34	1
crushed in heavy syrup	1 cup	199	1	19	12	35	1

FOOD	PORTION	CAL	PRO	VIT C	FOL	CA	IR
slices in heavy syrup	1 slice	45	tr	4	3	8	tr
slices in light syrup	1 slice	30	tr	4	3	8	tr
slices juice pack	1 slice	35	tr	6	–	8	tr
slices water pack	1 slice	19	tr	5	3	9	tr
tidbits in heavy syrup	1 cup	199	1	19	12	35	1
tidbits in juice	1 cup	150	1	24	–	34	1
tidbits in water	1 cup	79	1	19	12	37	1
FRESH							
pineapple; diced	1 cup	77	1	24	16	11	1
slice	1 slice	42	tr	13	9	6	tr
FROZEN							
chunks sweetened	½ cup	104	tr	10	–	11	tr
JUICE							
canned	1 cup	139	1	27	58	42	1
frzn; not prep	6 oz	387	3	91	–	84	2
frzn; as prep	1 cup	129	1	30	–	28	1

PINK BEANS

FOOD	PORTION	CAL	PRO	VIT C	FOL	CA	IR
DRIED							
cooked	1 cup	252	15	0	284	88	4
raw	1 cup	721	44	0	973	273	14

PINTO BEANS

FOOD	PORTION	CAL	PRO	VIT C	FOL	CA	IR
CANNED							
pinto	1 cup	186	11	2	145	89	4
DRIED							
cooked	1 cup	235	14	4	294	82	4
raw	1 cup	656	40	14	977	233	11
FROZEN							
cooked	3 oz	152	9	1	–	49	3
SPROUTS							
cooked	3½ oz	22	–	–	–	15	–
raw	3½ oz	62	–	–	–	43	–

FOOD	PORTION	CAL	PRO	VIT C	FOL	CA	IR
PISTACHIOS							
dried	1 oz	164	6	–	17	38	2
dried	1 cup	739	26	–	74	173	9
dry roasted	1 oz	172	4	–	–	20	1
dry roasted, salted	1 oz	172	4	–	–	20	1
dry roasted, salted	1 cup	776	19	–	–	90	4
PITANGA							
fresh	1	2	tr	2	–	1	tr
fresh	1 cup	57	1	46	–	16	tr
PIZZA							
TAKE-OUT							
cheese	⅛ of 12″ pie	140	8	1	59	116	1
cheese	12″ pie	1121	61	10	470	929	5
cheese, meat & vegetables	⅛ of 12″ pie	184	13	2	27	101	2
cheese, meat & vegetables	12″ pie	1472	104	13	215	805	12
pepperoni	⅛ of 12″ pie	181	10	2	53	65	1
pepperoni	12″ pie	1445	81	13	421	517	7
PLANTAINS							
FRESH							
sliced; cooked	½ cup	89	1	8	20	2	tr
uncooked	1	218	2	33	39	5	1
PLUMS							
CANNED							
purple in heavy syrup	3	119	tr	1	3	12	1
purple in heavy syrup	1 cup	320	1	1	7	24	2
purple in light syrup	3	83	tr	1	3	13	1

FOOD	PORTION	CAL	PRO	VIT C	FOL	CA	IR
purple in light syrup	1 cup	158	1	1	6	24	2
purple juice pack	3	55	tr	3	–	9	tr
purple juice pack	1 cup	146	1	7	–	25	1
purple water pack	3	39	tr	3	3	6	tr
purple water pack	1 cup	102	1	8	7	17	tr
FRESH							
plum	1	36	1	6	1	2	tr
sliced	1 cup	91	1	16	4	6	tr

POI

poi	½ cup	134	tr	5	–	19	1

POKEBERRY SHOOTS

FOOD	PORTION	CAL	PRO	VIT C	FOL	CA	IR
FRESH							
cooked	½ cup	16	2	67	–	43	1
raw	½ cup	18	2	109	–	42	1

POLLOCK

FOOD	PORTION	CAL	PRO	VIT C	FOL	CA	IR
Atlantic, raw	3 oz	78	17	–	–	51	tr
walleye, raw	3 oz	68	15	–	3	4	tr
walleye; cooked	1 fillet (2.1 oz)	68	14	–	2	4	tr
walleye; cooked	3 oz	96	20	–	3	5	tr

POMEGRANATES

pomegranates	1	104	1	9	–	5	tr

POMPANO

FOOD	PORTION	CAL	PRO	VIT C	FOL	CA	IR
Florida, raw	3 oz	140	16	–	–	19	1
Florida; cooked	3 oz	179	20	–	–	36	1

FOOD	PORTION	CAL	PRO	VIT C	FOL	CA	IR
POPCORN							
air-popped	1 cup	30	1	0	–	1	tr
popped w/ vegetable oil	1 cup	55	1	0	–	3	tr
sugar syrup coated	1 cup	135	2	0	–	2	1
POPPY SEEDS							
poppy seeds	1 tsp	15	1	–	–	41	0
PORK							
FRESH							
blade chop; roasted	1 (3.1 oz)	321	19	tr	4	11	1
center loin chop; broiled	1 (3.1 oz)	275	24	tr	4	4	1
center loin; roasted	3 oz	259	22	tr	1	5	1
loin w/ fat; roasted	3 oz	271	20	tr	4	7	1
shoulder, whole; roasted	3 oz	277	19	tr	4	6	1
spareribs; braised	3 oz	338	26	–	4	40	2
tenderloin, lean only; roasted	3 oz	141	24	tr	5	7	1
POT PIE							
HOME RECIPE							
beef; baked	⅓ of 9" pie (7.4 oz)	515	21	6	–	29	4
chicken	⅓ of 9" pie (8.1 oz)	545	23	5	–	70	3
POTATO							
CANNED							
potatoes	½ cup	54	1	5	6	5	1
FRESH							
baked w/ skin	1 (6½ oz)	220	5	26	22	20	3
baked w/o skin	1 (5 oz)	145	3	20	14	8	1

FOOD	PORTION	CAL	PRO	VIT C	FOL	CA	IR
baked w/o skin	½ cup	57	1	8	6	3	tr
baked, skin only	1 skin (2 oz)	115	2	8	–	20	4
boiled	½ cup	68	1	10	8	4	tr
microwaved	1 (7 oz)	212	5	31	24	22	3
microwaved w/o skin	½ cup	78	2	12	10	4	tr
raw w/o skin	1 (3.9 oz)	88	2	22	14	8	1
FROZEN french fries, thick cut; as prep	10 strips	109	2	5	9	5	1
french fries; as prep	10 strips	111	2	6	8	4	1
hashed brown; as prep	½ cup	170	2	5	–	12	1
potato puffs; as prep	½ cup	138	2	4	10	19	1
potato puffs; as prep	1 puff	16	tr	1	1	2	tr
HOME RECIPE au gratin	½ cup	160	6	12	10	146	1
hash brown	½ cup	163	2	5	6	6	1
mashed	½ cup	111	2	6	0	27	tr
o'brien	1 cup	157	5	32	16	70	1
potato dumpling	3½ oz	334	7	–	–	–	–
potato pancakes	1 (2.7 oz)	495	5	tr	22	21	1
scalloped	½ cup	105	4	13	10	70	1
MIX au gratin; as prep	4½ oz	127	3	4	–	114	tr
instant mashed flakes; as prep	½ cup	118	2	10	8	52	tr
instant mashed granules; as prep	½ cup	137	2	1	7	57	4
instant mashed granules; not prep	½ cup	80	2	10	7	13	tr
scalloped; as prep	4½ oz	127	3	5	2	49	1

FOOD	PORTION	CAL	PRO	VIT C	FOL	CA	IR
TAKE-OUT							
baked, topped w/ cheese sauce	1	475	15	26	28	310	3
baked, topped w/ cheese sauce, bacon	1	451	18	29	28	309	3
baked, topped w/ cheese sauce, broccoli	1	402	14	49	61	334	3
baked, topped w/ cheese sauce, chili	1	481	23	32	50	–	409
baked, topped w/ sour cream, chives	1	394	7	34	32	105	3
french fried; as prep in vegetable oil	1 reg	235	3	4	25	12	1
french fried; as prep in vegetable oil	1 lg	355	5	6	38	18	2
french fried; as prep in beef tallow	1 reg	237	3	4	25	12	1
french fried; as prep in beef tallow	1 lg	358	5	6	38	18	2
hash brown	½ cup	151	–	6	8	7	tr
mashed w/ whole milk, margarine	⅓ cup	66	2	tr	7	17	tr
salad	½ cup	179	3	13	8	24	1
salad	⅓ cup	108	1	1	24	13	tr

POTATO STARCH

FOOD	PORTION	CAL	PRO	VIT C	FOL	CA	IR
potato starch	3½ oz	335	1	0	–	35	2

POUT

FOOD	PORTION	CAL	PRO	VIT C	FOL	CA	IR
FRESH							
ocean, raw	3 oz	67	14	–	–	8	tr

PRETZELS

FOOD	PORTION	CAL	PRO	VIT C	FOL	CA	IR
sticks	10	10	tr	0	–	1	tr

FOOD	PORTION	CAL	PRO	VIT C	FOL	CA	IR
twist	1 (½ oz)	65	2	0	–	4	tr
twists, thin	10 (2 oz)	240	6	0	–	16	1

PRICKLY PEAR

fresh	1	42	1	14	–	58	tr

PRUNES

CANNED
in heavy syrup	5	90	1	2	–	15	tr
in heavy syrup	1 cup	245	2	7	–	40	1

DRIED
cooked w/ sugar	½ cup	147	1	3	tr	25	1
cooked w/o sugar	½ cup	113	1	3	tr	24	1
dried	10	201	2	3	3	43	2
dried	1 cup	385	4	5	6	82	4

JUICE
canned	1 cup	181	2	11	1	30	3

PUDDING

HOME RECIPE
corn	⅔ cup	181	7	5	42	67	1

MIX WITH WHOLE MILK
chocolate, instant	½ cup	155	4	1	–	130	tr
chocolate, regular	½ cup	150	4	1	–	146	tr
rice	½ cup	155	4	1	–	133	1
tapioca	½ cup	145	4	1	–	131	tr
vanilla, instant	½ cup	150	4	1	–	129	tr
vanilla, regular	½ cup	145	4	1	–	132	tr

PUMMELO

fresh	1	228	5	372	–	23	1
sections	1 cup	71	1	116	–	7	tr

FOOD	PORTION	CAL	PRO	VIT C	FOL	CA	IR
PUMPKIN							
CANNED							
pumpkin	½ cup	41	1	5	15	32	2
FRESH							
cooked, mashed	½ cup	24	1	5	15	32	2
flowers, raw	1	0	tr	1	–	1	tr
flowers; cooked	½ cup	10	1	3	–	25	1
leaves, raw	½ cup	4	1	2	–	8	tr
leaves; cooked	½ cup	7	1	tr	–	15	1
raw; cubed	½ cup	15	1	5	–	12	tr
SEEDS							
roasted	1 cup	1184	75	–	–	97	34
roasted	1 oz	148	9	–	–	12	4
salted & roasted	1 cup	1184	75	–	–	97	34
salted & roasted	1 oz	148	9	–	–	12	4
seeds, dried	1 oz	154	7	–	–	12	4
RADISHES							
FRESH							
chinese, raw	1 (12 oz)	62	2	74	–	91	1
chinese, raw; sliced	½ cup	8	tr	10	–	12	tr
chinese; sliced, cooked	½ cup	13	tr	11	–	12	tr
daikon, raw	1 (12 oz)	62	2	74	–	91	1
daikon, raw; sliced	½ cup	8	tr	10	–	12	tr
daikon; sliced, cooked	½ cup	13	tr	11	–	12	tr
red, raw	10	7	tr	10	12	9	tr
red, sliced	½ cup	10	tr	13	16	12	tr
white icicle, raw; sliced	½ cup	7	1	15	7	14	tr
SPROUTS							
raw	½ cup	8	1	6	18	10	tr

FOOD	PORTION	CAL	PRO	VIT C	FOL	CA	IR
RAISINS							
golden seedless	1 cup	437	5	5	5	76	3
seedless	1 cup	434	5	5	5	71	3
seedless	1 tbsp	27	tr	–	–	–	–
RASPBERRIES							
CANNED in heavy syrup	½ cup	117	1	11	13	14	1
FRESH raspberries	1 cup	61	1	31	–	27	1
raspberries	1 pint	154	3	78	–	69	2
FROZEN sweetened	1 cup	256	2	41	65	38	2
sweetened	1 pkg (10 oz)	291	2	47	74	43	2
RELISH							
cranberry orange	½ cup	246	tr	25	–	15	tr
sweet	1 tbsp	20	tr	1	–	3	tr
RHUBARB							
fresh	½ cup	13	1	5	4	52	tr
frzn	½ cup	60	tr	3	6	132	tr
frzn; as prep w/ sugar	½ cup	139	tr	4	6	174	tr
RICE							
BROWN long-grain, raw	½ cup	340	7	0	18	21	1
long-grain; cooked	½ cup	109	3	0	4	10	tr
medium-grain, raw	½ cup	344	7	0	19	31	2
medium-grain; cooked	½ cup	109	2	0	4	10	tr

FOOD	PORTION	CAL	PRO	VIT C	FOL	CA	IR
WHITE							
glutinous, raw	½ cup	341	6	0	6	10	1
glutinous; cooked	½ cup	116	2	0	1	2	tr
long-grain, instant, dry	½ cup	182	4	–	3	8	2
long-grain, instant; cooked	½ cup	80	2	0	3	6	tr
long-grain, parboiled, dry	½ cup	341	6	0	15	56	3
long-grain, parboiled; cooked	½ cup	100	2	0	3	17	tr
long-grain, raw	½ cup	336	7	0	8	26	4
long-grain; cooked	½ cup	131	3	0	3	12	1
medium-grain, raw	½ cup	353	6	0	9	9	4
medium-grain; cooked	½ cup	132	2	0	2	3	2
short-grain, raw	½ cup	358	7	0	6	3	4
short-grain; cooked	½ cup	133	2	0	2	1	1
starch	3½ oz	343	1	–	–	20	–
ROCKFISH							
FRESH							
Pacific, raw	3 oz	80	16	–	–	8	tr
Pacific; cooked	3 oz	103	20	–	–	10	tr
Pacific; cooked	1 fillet (5.2 oz)	180	36	–	–	18	1
ROE							
raw	1 oz	39	6	–	–	–	–
raw	3 oz	119	19	–	–	–	–
ROLL							
HOME RECIPE							
dinner	1 (1.2 oz)	120	3	0	–	16	1
READY-TO-EAT							
dinner	1 (1 oz)	85	2	tr	–	33	1

FOOD	PORTION	CAL	PRO	VIT C	FOL	CA	IR
frankfurter	1 (8/pkg)	115	3	tr	–	54	1
hamburger	1 (8/pkg)	115	3	tr	–	54	1
hard	1	155	5	0	–	24	1
submarine	1 (4.7 oz)	155	5	0	–	24	1

ROSE APPLE
fresh	3½ oz	32	1	22	–	20	1

ROSE HIP
fresh	3½ oz	91	4	1	–	257	1

ROSELLE
fresh	1 cup	28	1	7	–	123	1

ROSEMARY
dried	1 tsp	4	tr	1	–	15	tr

ROUGHY
FRESH orange, raw	3 oz	107	13	–	–	–	tr

RUTABAGA
cooked, mashed	½ cup	41	1	26	19	50	1
raw; cubed	½ cup	25	1	18	14	33	tr

SABLEFISH
raw	3 oz	166	11	–	–	–	tr
SMOKED sablefish	1 oz	72	5	–	–	–	–
sablefish	3 oz	218	15	–	–	–	–

SAFFLOWER
seeds, dried	1 oz	147	5	–	–	22	–

FOOD	PORTION	CAL	PRO	VIT C	FOL	CA	IR
SAFFRON							
saffron	1 tsp	2	tr	–	–	1	tr
SAGE							
ground	1 tsp	2	tr	tr	–	12	tr
SALAD							
TAKE-OUT							
tossed, w/o dressing	1½ cups	32	3	48	77	26	1
tossed, w/o dressing	¾ cup	16	1	24	39	13	tr
tossed, w/o dressing, w/ cheese & egg	1½ cups	102	9	10	85	100	tr
tossed, w/o dressing, w/ chicken	1½ cups	105	17	17	67	37	1
tossed, w/o dressing, w/ pasta & seafood	1½ cups	380	16	38	100	73	3
tossed, w/o dressing, w/ shrimp	1½ cups	107	15	9	87	60	tr
SALAD DRESSING							
HOME RECIPE							
french	1 tbsp	88	0	tr	–	1	0
vinegar & oil	1 tbsp	72	0	–	–	–	–
READY-TO-USE							
blue cheese	1 tbsp	77	1	tr	–	12	0
french	1 tbsp	67	tr	–	–	2	tr
italian	1 tbsp	69	tr	–	–	1	0
russian	1 tbsp	76	tr	1	–	3	tr
sesame seed	1 tbsp	68	1	–	–	–	–
thousand island	1 tbsp	59	tr	–	–	2	tr
READY-TO-USE REDUCED CALORIE							
french	1 tbsp	22	0	–	–	2	tr

FOOD	PORTION	CAL	PRO	VIT C	FOL	CA	IR
italian	1 tbsp	16	tr	–	–	0	0
russian	1 tbsp	23	tr	–	–	3	tr
thousand island	1 tbsp	24	tr	–	–	2	tr

SALMON
CANNED
chum w/ bone	3 oz	120	18	–	–	212	–
chum w/ bone	1 can (13.9 oz)	521	79	–	–	920	–
pink w/ bone	3 oz	118	17	0	13	181	1
pink w/ bone	1 can (15.9 oz)	631	90	0	70	969	4
sockeye w/ bone	3 oz	130	17	0	8	203	1
sockeye w/ bone	1 can (12.9 oz)	566	76	0	36	883	4

FRESH
atlantic, raw	3 oz	121	17	–	–	10	1
chinook, raw	3 oz	153	17	–	–	19	1
chum, raw	3 oz	102	17	–	–	9	tr
coho, raw	3 oz	124	18	1	–	–	1
coho; cooked	3 oz	157	23	1	–	–	1
coho; cooked	½ fillet (5.4 oz)	286	42	2	–	–	1
pink, raw	3 oz	99	17	–	–	–	1
sockeye, raw	3 oz	143	18	–	–	5	tr
sockeye; cooked	3 oz	183	23	–	–	6	1
sockeye; cooked	½ fillet (5.4 oz)	334	42	–	–	11	1

SMOKED
chinook	1 oz	33	5	–	1	3	tr
chinook	3 oz	99	16	–	2	9	1

FOOD	PORTION	CAL	PRO	VIT C	FOL	CA	IR
SALSIFY							
FRESH							
cooked, sliced	½ cup	46	2	3	–	32	tr
raw; sliced	½ cup	55	2	5	–	40	tr
SALT/SEASONED SALT							
salt	1 tsp	0	0	0	–	14	tr
SAPODILLA							
fresh	1	140	1	25	–	36	1
fresh; cut up	1 cup	199	1	35	–	51	2
SAPOTES							
fresh	1	301	5	45	–	88	2
SARDINES							
CANNED							
atlantic in oil w/ bone	1 can (3.2 oz)	192	23	–	11	351	3
atlantic in oil w/ bone	2	50	6	–	3	92	1
pacific in tomato sauce w/ bone	1 can (13 oz)	658	61	4	89	887	9
pacific in tomato sauce w/ bone	1	68	6	tr	9	91	1
FRESH							
raw	3½ oz	135	19	–	–	85	2
SAUCE							
DRY							
bearnaise; as prep w/ milk & butter	1 cup	701	8	–	–	–	–
cheese; as prep w/ milk	1 cup	307	16	2	–	570	tr
curry; as prep w/ milk	1 cup	270	11	–	–	485	–

FOOD	PORTION	CAL	PRO	VIT C	FOL	CA	IR
mushroom; as prep w/ milk	1 cup	228	11	–	–	–	–
sour cream; as prep w/ milk	1 cup	509	19	–	–	546	1
stroganoff; as prep	1 cup	271	12	–	–	521	1
sweet & sour; as prep	1 cup	294	1	–	–	41	2
teriyaki; as prep	1 cup	131	4	–	–	112	3
white; as prep w/ milk	1 cup	241	10	–	–	424	tr
JARRED barbecue	1 cup	188	5	18	–	48	2
teriyaki	1 tbsp	15	1	0	4	4	tr
teriyaki	1 oz	30	2	0	7	9	1

SAUERKRAUT

FOOD	PORTION	CAL	PRO	VIT C	FOL	CA	IR
CANNED canned	½ cup	22	1	17	–	36	2

SAUSAGE

FOOD	PORTION	CAL	PRO	VIT C	FOL	CA	IR
blutwurst, uncooked	3½ oz	424	13	–	–	7	6
bockwurst, pork & veal, raw	1 link (2.3 oz)	200	9	–	–	–	–
bockwurst, pork & veal, raw	1 oz	87	4	–	–	–	–
bratwurst, pork; cooked	1 link (3 oz)	256	12	1	–	38	1
bratwurst, pork; cooked	1 oz	85	4	0	–	13	tr
brotwurst, pork	1 oz	92	4	8	–	14	tr
brotwurst, pork & beef	1 link (2.5 oz)	226	10	20	–	34	1
country-style, pork; cooked	1 patty (1 oz)	100	5	1	–	9	tr
country-style, pork; cooked	1 link (½ oz)	48	3	tr	–	4	tr

FOOD	PORTION	CAL	PRO	VIT C	FOL	CA	IR
gelbwurst, uncooked	3½ oz	363	12	–	–	–	–
italian, pork, raw	1 (3 oz)	315	13	2	–	16	1
italian, pork, raw	1 (4 oz)	391	16	3	–	20	1
italian, pork; cooked	1 (2.4 oz)	216	13	1	–	16	1
italian, pork; cooked	1 (3 oz)	268	17	1	–	20	1
kielbasa, pork	1 oz	88	8	6	–	12	tr
knockwurst, pork & beef	1 (2.4 oz)	209	8	18	–	7	1
knockwurst, pork & beef	1 oz	87	3	8	–	3	tr
mettwurst, uncooked	3½ oz	483	13	–	–	13	2
plockwurst, uncooked	3½ oz	312	19	–	–	–	–
polish, pork	1 (8 oz)	739	32	2	–	26	3
polish, pork	1 oz	92	4	0	–	3	tr
pork & beef; cooked	1 patty (1 oz)	107	4	–	–	–	tr
pork & beef; cooked	1 link (½ oz)	52	2	–	–	–	tr
pork, country-style, raw	1 patty (2 oz)	238	–	–	–	10	–
pork, country-style, raw	1 link (1 oz)	118	–	–	–	5	–
pork, raw	1 patty (2 oz)	238	7	1	2	10	1
pork, raw	1 link (1 oz)	118	3	0	1	5	tr
pork; cooked	1 patty (1 oz)	100	5	0	–	9	tr
pork; cooked	1 link (½ oz)	48	3	0	–	4	tr
regensburger, uncooked	3½ oz	354	13	–	–	–	–
smoked, beef; cooked	1 sausage (1.4 oz)	134	–	–	–	4	–

FOOD	PORTION	CAL	PRO	VIT C	FOL	CA	IR
smoked, pork	1 link (2.4 oz)	256	15	1	–	20	1
smoked, pork	1 sm link (½ oz)	62	4	0	–	5	tr
smoked, pork & beef	1 link (2.4 oz)	229	9	3	–	7	tr
smoked, pork & beef	1 sm link (½ oz)	54	2	3	–	2	tr
vienna, canned	1 (1½ oz)	45	2	0	–	2	tr
vienna, canned	7 (4 oz)	315	12	0	–	12	1
weisswurst, uncooked	3½ oz	305	11	–	–	25	–
TAKE-OUT							
pork	1 patty (1 oz)	100	5	0	–	9	tr
pork	1 link (.5 oz)	48	3	0	–	4	tr

SAVORY

ground	1 tsp	4	tr	–	–	30	1

SCALLOP

FRESH							
raw	3 oz	75	14	–	–	21	tr
HOME RECIPE							
breaded & fried	2 lg	67	6	–	–	13	tr
TAKE-OUT							
breaded & fried	6 (5 oz)	386	16	0	40	18	2

SCUP

FRESH							
raw	3 oz	89	16	–	–	34	tr

SEAWEED

DRIED							
agar	1 oz	87	2	0	–	78	6
spirulina	1 oz	83	16	3	–	–	8

FOOD	PORTION	CAL	PRO	VIT C	FOL	CA	IR
FRESH							
agar	1 oz	tr	tr	0	–	15	1
irishmoss	1 oz	14	tr	–	–	21	3
kelp	1 oz	12	tr	–	51	48	1
kombu	1 oz	12	tr	–	51	48	1
laver	1 oz	10	2	11	–	20	1
nori	1 oz	10	2	11	–	20	1
spirulina	1 oz	7	2	tr	–	–	–
tangle	1 oz	12	tr	–	51	48	1
wakame	1 oz	13	1	1	–	43	1
SEMOLINA							
dry	½ cup	303	11	0	61	14	4
SESAME							
seeds	1 tsp	16	1	–	–	4	tr
seeds, dried	1 tbsp	52	2	0	9	88	1
seeds, dried	1 cup	825	26	0	139	1404	21
seeds, roasted & toasted	1 oz	161	14	–	–	281	4
sesame butter	1 tbsp	95	3	0	–	154	3
tahini from roasted & toasted kernels	1 tbsp	89	3	0	–	64	1
tahini from stone ground kernels	1 tbsp	86	3	0	–	63	tr
tahini from unroasted kernels	1 tbsp	85	3	–	–	20	1
SESBANIA							
flower	1	1	tr	2	–	1	tr
flowers	1 cup	5	tr	15	–	4	tr
flowers; cooked	1 cup	23	1	39	–	23	1

FOOD	PORTION	CAL	PRO	VIT C	FOL	CA	IR
SHAD							
FRESH							
american, raw	3 oz	167	14	–	–	40	1
SHALLOTS							
DRIED							
dried	1 tbsp	3	tr	tr	1	2	tr
FRESH							
raw; chopped	1 tbsp	7	tr	1	–	4	tr
SHARK							
batter-dipped & fried	3 oz	194	16	–	–	52	1
raw	3 oz	111	18	–	–	29	1
SHEEPSHEAD FISH							
cooked	1 fillet (6.5 oz)	234	48	–	–	70	1
cooked	3 oz	107	22	–	–	32	1
raw	3 oz	92	17	–	–	18	tr
SHELLFISH SUBSTITUTES							
crab, imitation	3 oz	87	10	–	–	11	tr
scallop, imitation	3 oz	84	11	–	–	7	tr
shrimp, imitation	3 oz	86	11	–	–	16	1
surimi	1 oz	28	4	–	–	2	tr
surimi	3 oz	84	13	–	–	7	tr
SHELLIE BEANS							
CANNED							
shellie beans	½ cup	37	2	4	–	36	1
SHRIMP							
canned	1 cup	154	30	–	2	75	4
canned	3 oz	102	20	–	2	50	2

FOOD	PORTION	CAL	PRO	VIT C	FOL	CA	IR
FRESH							
cooked	4 large	22	5	–	1	9	1
cooked	3 oz	84	18	–	3	33	3
raw	3 oz	90	17	–	3	44	2
raw	4 large	30	6	–	1	15	1
HOME RECIPE							
breaded & fried	3 oz	206	18	–	7	57	1
breaded & fried	4 large	73	6	–	2	20	tr
TAKE-OUT							
breaded & fried	6 to 8 (6 oz)	454	19	0	48	84	3

SMELT

FOOD	PORTION	CAL	PRO	VIT C	FOL	CA	IR
FRESH							
rainbow, raw	3 oz	83	15	–	–	51	1
rainbow; cooked	3 oz	106	19	–	–	65	1

SNAP BEANS

FOOD	PORTION	CAL	PRO	VIT C	FOL	CA	IR
CANNED							
green	½ cup	13	1	3	22	18	1
yellow	½ cup	13	1	3	22	18	1
FRESH							
green, raw	½ cup	17	1	9	20	21	1
green, raw	½ cup	17	1	9	20	21	1
green; cooked	½ cup	22	1	6	21	29	1
yellow, raw	½ cup	17	1	9	20	21	1
yellow; cooked	½ cup	22	1	6	21	29	1
FROZEN							
cooked	½ cup	18	1	6	–	31	1
yellow; cooked	½ cup	18	1	6	–	31	1

FOOD	PORTION	CAL	PRO	VIT C	FOL	CA	IR
SNAPPER							
FRESH							
cooked	1 fillet (6 oz)	217	45	–	–	69	tr
cooked	3 oz	109	22	–	–	34	tr
raw	3 oz	85	17	–	–	27	tr
SODA							
club	12 oz	0	0	0	0	17	–
cola	12 oz	151	tr	0	0	9	tr
cream	12 oz	191	0	0	0	19	tr
diet cola	12 oz	2	tr	0	0	12	tr
diet cola w/ nutrasweet	12 oz	2	tr	0	0	12	tr
diet cola w/ saccharin	12 oz	2	tr	0	0	14	tr
ginger ale	12 oz can	124	tr	0	0	12	tr
grape	12 oz	161	0	0	0	12	tr
lemon lime	12 oz	149	0	0	0	9	tr
orange	12 oz	177	0	0	0	19	tr
pepper type	12 oz	151	0	0	0	12	tr
quinine	12 oz	125	0	0	0	5	–
root beer	12 oz	152	tr	0	0	19	tr
tonic water	12 oz	125	0	0	0	5	–
SOLE							
FRESH							
lemon, raw	3½ oz	85	17	–	–	–	–
raw	3½ oz	90	18	0	–	29	1
SORGHUM							
sorghum	½ cup	325	11	0	–	27	4

FOOD	PORTION	CAL	PRO	VIT C	FOL	CA	IR
SOUFFLE							
HOME RECIPE							
spinach souffle	1 cup	218	11	3	62	230	1
SOUP							
CANNED							
asparagus, cream of; as prep w/ milk	1 cup	161	6	4	–	175	1
asparagus, cream of; as prep w/ water	1 cup	87	1	3	–	29	1
bean black; as prep w/ water	1 cup	116	6	1	25	45	2
beef broth, ready-to-serve	1 can (14 oz)	27	5	0	–	25	1
beef broth, ready-to-serve	1 cup	16	3	0	–	15	tr
beef noodle; as prep w/ water	1 cup	84	5	tr	4	15	1
black bean turtle soup	1 cup	218	14	6	146	84	5
celery, cream of; as prep w/ milk	1 cup	165	6	1	9	186	1
celery, cream of; as prep w/ water	1 cup	90	2	tr	2	40	1
celery, cream of; not prep	1 can (10¾ oz)	219	4	1	6	98	2
cheese; as prep w/ milk	1 cup	230	9	1	–	288	1
cheese; as prep w/ water	1 cup	155	5	0	–	142	1
cheese; not prep	1 can (11 oz)	377	13	0	–	345	2
chicken vegetable; as prep w/ water	1 cup	74	4	1	–	18	1
chicken broth; as prep w/ water	1 cup	39	5	0	–	9	1
chicken cream of; as prep w/ milk	1 cup	191	7	1	8	180	1

FOOD	PORTION	CAL	PRO	VIT C	FOL	CA	IR
chicken cream of; as prep w/ water	1 cup	116	3	tr	2	34	1
chicken gumbo; as prep w/ water	1 cup	56	3	5	–	24	1
chicken noodle; as prep w/ water	1 cup	75	4	tr	2	17	1
chicken rice; as prep w/ water	1 cup	251	4	tr	1	17	1
clam chowder, Manhattan; as prep w/ water	1 cup	78	4	3	10	34	2
clam chowder, New England; as prep w/ milk	1 cup	163	9	4	10	187	1
clam chowder, New England; as prep w/ water	1 cup	95	5	2	4	43	1
consomme w/ gelatin; as prep w/ water	1 cup	29	5	1	3	8	1
consomme w/ gelatin; not prep	1 can (10½ oz)	71	13	2	7	21	1
escarole, ready-to-serve	1 cup	27	2	–	–	32	1
french onion; as prep w/ water	1 cup	57	4	1	15	26	1
gazpacho, ready-to-serve	1 cup	57	9	3	–	24	1
minestrone; as prep w/ water	1 cup	83	4	1	16	34	1
mushroom, cream of; as prep w/ milk	1 cup	203	6	2	–	178	1
mushroom, cream of; as prep w/ water	1 cup	129	2	1	–	46	1
oyster stew; as prep w/ milk	1 cup	134	6	4	–	167	1
oyster stew; as prep w/ water	1 cup	59	2	3	–	22	1
pepperpot; as prep w/ water	1 cup	103	6	1	tr	23	1

FOOD	PORTION	CAL	PRO	VIT C	FOL	CA	IR
potato, cream of; as prep w/ milk	1 cup	148	6	1	9	166	1
potato, cream of; as prep w/ water	1 cup	73	2	0	3	20	tr
scotch broth; as prep w/ water	1 cup	80	5	1	–	15	1
split pea w/ ham; as prep w/ water	1 cup	189	10	1	3	22	2
tomato; as prep w/ milk	1 cup	160	6	68	21	159	2
tomato; as prep w/ water	1 cup	86	2	67	15	13	2
vegetarian vegetable; as prep w/ water	1 cup	72	2	1	11	21	1
vichyssoise	1 cup	148	6	1	9	166	1
DRY							
asparagus, cream of; as prep w/ water	1 cup	59	2	–	–	–	–
beef broth; as prep w/ water	1 cup	19	1	–	–	5	–
beef broth; as prep w/ water	1 cube + 1 cup water	8	1	–	–	–	tr
beef broth; not prep	1 pkg (.2 oz)	14	1	–	–	4	–
beef broth; not prep	1 cube (3.6 g)	6	1	–	–	–	tr
celery, cream of; as prep w/ water	1 cup	63	3	–	–	–	–
chicken broth cube; as prep w/ water	1 cup	13	1	–	–	–	tr
chicken broth; as prep w/ water	1 cup	21	1	tr	–	15	tr
chicken broth; not prep	1 pkg (.2 oz)	16	1	tr	–	11	tr
chicken broth; not prep	1 cube (4.8 g)	9	1	–	–	–	tr

FOOD	PORTION	CAL	PRO	VIT C	FOL	CA	IR
chicken cream of; as prep w/ water	1 cup	107	2	–	–	76	–
chicken noodle; as prep w/ water	1 cup	53	3	tr	1	32	1
french onion; not prep	1 pkg (1.4 oz)	115	5	1	6	55	1
leek; as prep w/ water	1 cup	71	2	–	–	–	–
onion; as prep w/ water	1 cup	28	1	tr	2	13	tr
onion; not prep	1 pkg (1.4 oz)	115	5	1	6	55	1
tomato; as prep w/ water	1 cup	102	2	5	7	54	tr
HOME RECIPE black bean turtle soup	1 cup	241	15	0	158	103	5

SOUR CREAM

REGULAR

sour cream	1 tbsp	26	tr	tr	1	14	tr
sour cream	1 cup	493	7	2	25	268	tr

SOUR CREAM SUBSTITUTES

nondairy	1 oz	59	1	0	0	1	–
nondairy	1 cup	479	6	0	0	6	–

SOURSOP

fresh	1	416	6	129	–	88	4
fresh; cut up	1 cup	150	2	46	–	32	1

SOY

lecithin	1 tbsp	120	0	–	–	–	–
milk	1 cup	79	7	0	4	10	1
soy sauce	1 tbsp	7	tr	0	2	1	tr
soy sauce, shoyu	1 tbsp	9	1	0	3	3	tr

FOOD	PORTION	CAL	PRO	VIT C	FOL	CA	IR
soy sauce, tamari	1 tbsp	11	2	0	3	4	tr
soybean sprouts, raw	½ cup	45	5	5	60	24	1
soybean sprouts; cooked	½ cup	38	4	4	–	28	1
soybeans, dry roasted	½ cup	387	34	4	176	232	3
soybeans, roasted	½ cup	405	30	2	182	119	3
soybeans, roasted & toasted	1 oz	129	11	1	64	39	1
soybeans, roasted & toasted	1 cup	490	40	2	244	149	5
soybeans, salted, roasted & toasted	1 oz	129	11	1	64	39	1
soybeans, salted, roasted & toasted	1 cup	490	40	2	244	149	5
soybeans, dried	1 cup	774	68	11	698	515	29
soybeans; cooked	1 cup	298	29	3	93	175	9

SPAGHETTI SAUCE

JARRED
| marinara sauce | 1 cup | 171 | 4 | 32 | – | 44 | 2 |
| spaghetti sauce | 1 cup | 272 | 12 | 28 | – | 70 | 2 |

SPINACH

CANNED
| spinach | ½ cup | 25 | 3 | 15 | 105 | 135 | 2 |

FRESH
cooked	½ cup	21	3	9	131	122	3
mustard, raw; chopped	½ cup	17	2	98	–	158	1
mustard; chopped, cooked	½ cup	14	2	59	–	142	1
new zealand, raw	½ cup	4	tr	8	–	16	tr
new zealand; chopped, cooked	½ cup	11	1	14	–	43	1
raw; chopped	½ cup	6	1	8	54	28	1

FOOD	PORTION	CAL	PRO	VIT C	FOL	CA	IR
raw; chopped	1 pkg (10 oz)	46	6	57	397	202	6
FROZEN cooked	½ cup	27	3	12	102	139	1
JUICE spinach juice	3½ oz	7	1	29	–	1	–

SPOT

FOOD	PORTION	CAL	PRO	VIT C	FOL	CA	IR
FRESH raw	3 oz	105	16	–	–	12	tr

SQUAB

FOOD	PORTION	CAL	PRO	VIT C	FOL	CA	IR
breast w/o skin, raw	1 (3.5 oz)	135	22	–	–	–	–
w/ skin, raw	1 squab (6.9 oz)	584	37	–	–	–	–
w/o skin, raw	1 squab (5.9 oz)	239	29	–	–	–	–

SQUASH

FOOD	PORTION	CAL	PRO	VIT C	FOL	CA	IR
CANNED crookneck, sliced	½ cup	14	1	3	11	13	1
FRESH acorn; cooked, mashed	½ cup	41	1	8	14	32	1
acorn; cubed, baked	½ cup	57	1	11	19	45	1
butternut; baked	½ cup	41	1	15	20	42	1
crookneck, raw; sliced	½ cup	12	1	5	15	14	tr
crookneck; sliced, cooked	½ cup	18	1	5	18	24	tr
hubbard; baked	½ cup	51	3	10	17	17	tr
hubbard; cooked, mashed	½ cup	35	2	8	12	12	tr
scallop, raw; sliced	½ cup	12	1	12	20	12	tr
scallop; sliced, cooked	½ cup	14	1	10	19	14	tr
spaghetti; cooked	½ cup	23	1	3	6	17	tr

FOOD	PORTION	CAL	PRO	VIT C	FOL	CA	IR
FROZEN							
butternut; cooked, mashed	½ cup	47	1	4	–	23	1
crookneck, sliced; cooked	½ cup	24	1	7	12	19	tr
SEEDS							
dried	1 oz	154	7	–	–	12	4
dried	1 cup	747	34	–	–	59	21
roasted	1 oz	148	9	–	–	12	4
roasted	1 cup	1184	75	–	–	97	34
salted & roasted	1 oz	148	9	–	–	12	4
salted & roasted	1 cup	1184	75	–	–	97	34
whole, salted; roasted	1 oz	127	6	–	–	16	1
whole, salted; roasted	1 cup	285	12	–	–	35	2
whole; roasted	1 oz	127	5	–	–	16	1
whole; roasted	1 cup	285	12	–	–	35	2

SQUID

FOOD	PORTION	CAL	PRO	VIT C	FOL	CA	IR
FRESH							
fried	3 oz	149	15	4	–	33	1
raw	3 oz	78	13	4	–	27	1

SQUIRREL

FOOD	PORTION	CAL	PRO	VIT C	FOL	CA	IR
raw	1 oz	34	6	–	–	1	1
roasted	3 oz	116	21	–	–	2	5

STRAWBERRIES

FOOD	PORTION	CAL	PRO	VIT C	FOL	CA	IR
CANNED							
in heavy syrup	½ cup	117	1	40	36	16	1
FRESH							
strawberries	1 cup	45	1	85	26	21	1
strawberries	1 pint	97	2	182	57	45	1
FROZEN							
sweetened sliced	1 cup	245	1	106	38	29	1

FOOD	PORTION	CAL	PRO	VIT C	FOL	CA	IR
sweetened sliced	1 pkg (10 oz)	273	2	118	42	31	2
unsweetened	1 cup	52	1	61	25	23	1
whole sweetened	1 cup	200	1	101	10	29	1
whole sweetened	1 pkg (10 oz)	223	1	112	11	32	1

STUFFING/ DRESSING

MIX
bread, dry	1 cup	500	9	0	–	92	2

STURGEON

FRESH
cooked	3 oz	115	18	–	–	–	–
raw	3 oz	90	14	–	–	–	–

SMOKED
sturgeon	3 oz	147	27	–	–	–	–
sturgeon	1 oz	48	9	–	–	–	–

SUCKER

FRESH
white, raw	3 oz	79	14	–	–	60	1

SUGAR

brown	1 cup	820	0	0	–	187	5
powdered; sifted	1 cup	385	0	0	–	1	tr
white	1 cup	770	0	0	–	3	tr
white	1 tbsp	45	0	0	–	tr	tr
white	1 packet (6 g)	25	0	0	–	tr	tr

SUGAR-APPLE

fresh	1	146	3	66	–	37	1
fresh; cut up	1 cup	236	5	91	–	59	2

FOOD	PORTION	CAL	PRO	VIT C	FOL	CA	IR
SUNFISH							
FRESH							
pumpkinseed, raw	3 oz	76	16	–	–	68	1
SUNFLOWER SEEDS							
dried	1 oz	162	33	–	–	33	2
dried	1 cup	821	33	–	–	168	10
dry roasted	1 oz	165	5	–	–	20	1
dry roasted	1 cup	745	25	–	–	90	5
dry roasted, salted	1 oz	165	5	–	–	20	1
dry roasted, salted	1 cup	745	25	–	–	90	5
oil roasted	1 oz	175	6	tr	67	16	2
oil roasted	1 cup	830	29	2	316	76	9
oil roasted, salted	1 cup	830	29	2	316	76	9
oil roasted, salted	1 oz	175	6	tr	67	16	2
sunflower butter w/o salt	1 tbsp	93	3	tr	–	19	1
toasted	1 oz	176	5	–	–	16	2
toasted	1 cup	826	23	–	–	76	9
toasted, salted	1 oz	176	5	–	–	16	2
toasted, salted	1 cup	826	23	–	–	76	9
SWAMP CABBAGE							
FRESH							
chopped, cooked	½ cup	10	1	8	–	26	1
raw; chopped	1 cup	11	1	31	–	43	1
SWEET POTATO							
CANNED							
in syrup	½ cup	106	1	11	–	16	1
pieces	1 cup	183	3	53	33	44	2

FOOD	PORTION	CAL	PRO	VIT C	FOL	CA	IR
FRESH							
baked w/ skin	1 (3½ oz)	118	2	28	26	32	1
leaves; cooked	½ cup	11	1	1	–	8	tr
mashed	½ cup	172	3	28	18	35	1
FROZEN							
cooked	½ cup	88	2	8	20	31	tr
HOME RECIPE							
candied	3½ oz	144	1	7	12	27	1

SWEETBREADS

FOOD	PORTION	CAL	PRO	VIT C	FOL	CA	IR
beef; braised	3 oz	230	23	17	–	14	2
lamb; braised	3 oz	199	19	17	11	10	2
veal; braised	3 oz	218	25	5	–	–	2

SWISS CHARD

FOOD	PORTION	CAL	PRO	VIT C	FOL	CA	IR
FRESH							
cooked	½ cup	18	2	16	–	51	2
raw; chopped	½ cup	3	tr	5	–	9	tr

SWORDFISH

FOOD	PORTION	CAL	PRO	VIT C	FOL	CA	IR
cooked	3 oz	132	22	1	–	5	1
raw	3 oz	103	17	1	–	4	1

SYRUP

FOOD	PORTION	CAL	PRO	VIT C	FOL	CA	IR
corn	2 tbsp	122	0	0	–	1	tr
raspberry	3½ oz	267	tr	16	–	16	2

TAMARIND

FOOD	PORTION	CAL	PRO	VIT C	FOL	CA	IR
FRESH							
cut up	1 cup	287	3	4	–	89	3
tamarind	1	5	tr	tr	–	1	tr

FOOD	PORTION	CAL	PRO	VIT C	FOL	CA	IR
TANGERINE							
CANNED							
in light syrup	½ cup	76	1	25	–	9	tr
juice pack	½ cup	46	1	43	–	14	tr
FRESH							
sections	1 cup	86	1	60	40	27	tr
tangerine	1	37	1	26	17	12	tr
JUICE							
canned sweetened	1 cup	125	1	55	–	45	1
fresh	1 cup	106	1	77	–	44	tr
frzn sweetened, not prep	6 oz	344	3	182	35	57	1
frzn sweetened; as prep	1 cup	110	1	58	11	18	tr
TAPIOCA							
pearl, dry	⅓ cup	174	tr	0	2	10	tr
starch	3½ oz	344	58	0	–	12	1
TARO							
chips	10	110	tr	–	–	10	tr
chips	½ cup	57	tr	–	–	5	tr
leaves; cooked	½ cup	18	2	26	–	63	1
raw; sliced	½ cup	56	1	2	–	22	tr
shoots; sliced, cooked	½ cup	10	1	–	–	9	tr
sliced, cooked	½ cup	94	tr	3	–	12	tr
tahitian; sliced, cooked	½ cup	30	3	26	–	101	1
TARRAGON							
ground	1 tsp	5	tr	–	–	18	1
TEA/HERBAL TEA							
REGULAR							
brewed tea	6 oz	2	0	0	9	0	tr

FOOD	PORTION	CAL	PRO	VIT C	FOL	CA	IR
instant artificially sweetened, lemon flavored; as prep w/ water	8 oz	5	tr	0	5	5	tr
instant sweetened, lemon flavor; as prep w/ water	9 oz	87	tr	0	10	6	tr
instant unsweetened, lemon flavor; as prep w/ water	8 oz	4	tr	0	–	5	tr
instant unsweetened; as prep w/ water	8 oz	2	tr	0	1	5	tr

TEMPEH

FOOD	PORTION	CAL	PRO	VIT C	FOL	CA	IR
tempeh	½ cup	165	16	0	43	77	2

TEXTURED VEGETABLE PROTEIN

FOOD	PORTION	CAL	PRO	VIT C	FOL	CA	IR
simulated meat product	1 oz	88	11	–	–	57	3

THYME

FOOD	PORTION	CAL	PRO	VIT C	FOL	CA	IR
ground	1 tsp	4	tr	–	–	26	2

TILEFISH

FOOD	PORTION	CAL	PRO	VIT C	FOL	CA	IR
FRESH							
cooked	½ fillet (5.3 oz)	220	37	–	–	39	tr
cooked	3 oz	125	21	–	–	22	tr
raw	3 oz	81	15	–	–	22	tr

TOFU

FOOD	PORTION	CAL	PRO	VIT C	FOL	CA	IR
firm	¼ block (3 oz)	118	13	tr	24	166	8
fried	1 piece (½ oz)	35	2	0	4	48	1
fuyu, salted & fermented	1 block (⅓ oz)	13	1	–	–	5	tr

FOOD	PORTION	CAL	PRO	VIT C	FOL	CA	IR
koyadofu, dried, frozen	1 piece (½ oz)	82	8	tr	16	62	2
okara	½ cup	47	2	0	–	49	1
regular	¼ block (4 oz)	88	9	tr	17	122	6

TOMATO

CANNED

FOOD	PORTION	CAL	PRO	VIT C	FOL	CA	IR
red, whole	½ cup	24	1	18	–	32	1
stewed	½ cup	34	1	17	–	47	1
tomato paste	½ cup	110	5	55	–	46	4
tomato paste w/o salt	½ cup	110	5	55	–	46	4
tomato puree	1 cup	102	4	88	–	37	2
tomato puree w/o salt	1 cup	102	4	88	–	37	2
tomato sauce	½ cup	37	2	16	–	17	1
tomato sauce spanish style	½ cup	40	2	11	–	20	4
tomato sauce w/ mushrooms	½ cup	42	2	15	–	16	1
tomato sauce w/ onion	½ cup	52	1	16	–	20	1
tomatoes w/ green chilies	½ cup	18	1	8	–	24	tr
wedges in tomato juice	½ cup	34	1	19	–	34	1

FRESH

FOOD	PORTION	CAL	PRO	VIT C	FOL	CA	IR
cooked	½ cup	30	1	25	11	10	1
green	1	30	1	29	–	16	1
red	1	24	1	22	12	8	1
red; chopped	1 cup	35	2	32	17	12	1

HOME RECIPE

FOOD	PORTION	CAL	PRO	VIT C	FOL	CA	IR
stewed tomatoes	1 cup	59	2	15	11	19	1

JUICE

FOOD	PORTION	CAL	PRO	VIT C	FOL	CA	IR
beef broth & tomato	5½ oz	61	1	2	–	19	1
clam & tomato	1 can (5½ oz)	77	1	7	–	21	1

FOOD	PORTION	CAL	PRO	VIT C	FOL	CA	IR
tomato juice	6 fl oz	32	1	33	36	16	1
tomato juice	½ cup	21	1	22	24	10	1

TONGUE

FOOD	PORTION	CAL	PRO	VIT C	FOL	CA	IR
beef; simmered	3 oz	241	19	tr	4	6	3
lamb; braised	3 oz	234	18	6	2	8	2

TREE FERN

FOOD	PORTION	CAL	PRO	VIT C	FOL	CA	IR
chopped, cooked	½ cup	28	tr	21	–	6	tr

TRITICALE

FOOD	PORTION	CAL	PRO	VIT C	FOL	CA	IR
dry	½ cup	323	13	0	70	36	2
FRESH							
rainbow, raw	3 oz	100	17	3	–	57	2
rainbow; cooked	3 oz	129	22	3	–	73	2
seatrout, raw	3 oz	88	14	–	–	15	tr

TRUFFLES

FOOD	PORTION	CAL	PRO	VIT C	FOL	CA	IR
fresh	3½ oz	25	6	–	–	24	4

TUNA

FOOD	PORTION	CAL	PRO	VIT C	FOL	CA	IR
CANNED							
light in oil	3 oz	169	25	–	5	11	1
light in oil	1 can (6 oz)	399	50	–	9	23	2
light in water	1 can (5.8 oz)	216	49	–	6	20	5
light in water	3 oz	111	25	–	3	10	3
white in oil	3 oz	158	23	–	4	4	1
white in oil	1 can (6.2 oz)	331	47	–	8	8	1
white in water	1 can (6 oz)	234	46	–	7	–	1
white in water	3 oz	116	23	–	4	–	1

FOOD	PORTION	CAL	PRO	VIT C	FOL	CA	IR
FRESH							
bluefin, raw	3 oz	122	20	–	–	–	1
bluefin; cooked	3 oz	157	25	–	–	–	1
skipjack, raw	3 oz	88	19	–	–	24	1
yellowfin, raw	3 oz	92	20	–	–	14	1

TUNA DISHES

FOOD	PORTION	CAL	PRO	VIT C	FOL	CA	IR
TAKE-OUT							
tuna salad	3 oz	159	14	1	6	15	1
tuna salad	1 cup	383	33	5	15	35	2
tuna salad submarine sandwich w/ lettuce, oil	1	584	30	4	58	74	3

TURBOT

FOOD	PORTION	CAL	PRO	VIT C	FOL	CA	IR
FRESH							
european, raw	3 oz	81	14	–	–	15	–

TURKEY

FOOD	PORTION	CAL	PRO	VIT C	FOL	CA	IR
CANNED							
w/ broth	½ can (2.5 oz)	116	17	1	–	9	1
w/ broth	1 can (5 oz)	231	34	3	–	17	3
FRESH							
back w/ skin; roasted	½ back (9 oz)	637	70	0	21	87	6
breast w/ skin; roasted	4 oz	212	32	0	7	24	2
dark meat w/ skin; roasted	3.6 oz	230	29	0	9	34	2
dark meat w/o skin; roasted	3 oz	170	26	0	9	19	2
dark meat w/o skin; roasted	1 cup (5 oz)	262	40	0	13	45	3
leg w/ skin; roasted	2.5 oz	147	20	0	6	23	2
leg w/ skin; roasted	1 (1.2 lbs)	1133	152	0	49	176	13

FOOD	PORTION	CAL	PRO	VIT C	FOL	CA	IR
light meat w/ skin; roasted	4.7 oz	268	39	0	8	29	2
light meat w/ skin; roasted	from ½ turkey (2.3 lbs)	2069	87	0	61	225	15
light meat w/o skin; roasted	4 oz	183	35	0	7	23	2
neck, raw	1 (6.3 oz)	243	36	0	19	60	4
neck; simmered	1 (5.3 oz)	274	41	0	12	56	3
skin; roasted	1 oz	141	13	0	1	11	1
skin; roasted	from ½ turkey (9 oz)	1096	49	0	10	87	4
w/ skin, neck & giblets, raw	½ turkey (6 lbs)	4369	216	4	639	421	47
w/ skin, neck & giblets, raw	9 oz	533	25	tr	53	68	5
w/ skin, neck & giblets; roasted	½ turkey (8.8 lbs)	4123	190	1	409	525	40
w/ skin; roasted	½ turkey (4 lbs)	3857	522	0	130	488	33
w/ skin; roasted	8.4 oz	498	67	0	17	63	4
w/o skin; roasted	7.3 oz	354	61	0	16	52	4
w/o skin; roasted	1 cup (5 oz)	238	41	0	10	35	2
wing w/ skin; roasted	1 (6.5 oz)	426	51	0	10	44	3
FROZEN roast, boneless, seasoned, light & dark meat, raw	1 pkg (2.5 lbs)	1358	200	–	–	11	24
roast, boneless, seasoned, light & dark meat; roasted	1 pkg (1.7 lbs)	1213	167	–	–	40	13

FOOD	PORTION	CAL	PRO	VIT C	FOL	CA	IR
FROZEN PREPARED							
gravy & turkey	1 cup (8.4 oz)	160	14	–	–	33	2
gravy & turkey	1 pkg (5 oz)	95	8	–	–	20	1
READY-TO-USE							
bologna	1 oz	57	4	–	–	24	tr
breast	1 slice (¾ oz)	23	5	0	–	1	tr
diced, light & dark, seasoned	1 oz	39	5	–	–	0	1
diced, light & dark, seasoned	½ lb	313	42	–	–	2	4
ham, thigh meat	2 oz	73	11	–	–	5	2
ham, thigh meat	1 pkg (8 oz)	291	43	–	–	22	6
pastrami	2 oz	80	10	–	–	5	1
pastrami	1 pkg (8 oz)	320	42	–	–	20	4
patties; battered, fried	1 (3.3 oz)	266	13	–	–	13	2
patties; battered, fried	1 (2.3 oz)	181	9	–	–	9	1
patties; breaded, fried	1 (2.3 oz)	181	9	–	–	9	1
patties; breaded, fried	1 (3.3 oz)	266	13	–	–	13	2
poultry salad sandwich spread	1 tbsp	109	2	0	1	1	tr
poultry salad sandwich spread	1 oz	238	4	0	1	3	tr
prebasted breast w/ skin; roasted	1 breast (3.8 lbs)	2175	383	0	–	149	11
prebasted breast w/ skin; roasted	½ breast (1.9 lbs)	1087	191	0	–	75	6
prebasted thigh w/ skin; roasted	1 thigh (11 oz)	494	59	–	–	25	5
roll, light & dark meat	1 oz	42	5	–	–	9	tr

FOOD	PORTION	CAL	PRO	VIT C	FOL	CA	IR
roll, light meat	1 oz	42	5	–	–	11	tr
salami, cooked	2 oz	111	9	–	–	11	1
salami, cooked	1 pkg (8 oz)	446	37	–	–	44	4
turkey loaf, breast meat	2 slices (1.5 oz)	47	10	0	–	3	tr
turkey loaf, breast meat	1 pkg (6 oz)	187	38	0	–	12	1
turkey sticks; battered, fried	1 stick (2.3 oz)	178	9	–	–	9	1
turkey sticks; breaded, fried	1 stick (2.3 oz)	178	9	–	–	9	1

TURMERIC

FOOD	PORTION	CAL	PRO	VIT C	FOL	CA	IR
ground	1 tsp	8	tr	1	–	4	1

TURNIPS

FOOD	PORTION	CAL	PRO	VIT C	FOL	CA	IR
CANNED							
greens	½ cup	17	2	18	48	138	2
FRESH							
cooked, mashed	½ cup	21	1	13	11	26	tr
greens, raw; chopped	½ cup	7	tr	17	54	53	tr
greens; chopped, cooked	½ cup	15	1	20	85	99	1
raw; cubed	½ cup	18	1	14	10	20	tr
FROZEN							
greens; cooked	½ cup	24	3	18	32	125	2

TURTLE

FOOD	PORTION	CAL	PRO	VIT C	FOL	CA	IR
raw	3½ oz	85	18	–	–	107	2

TUSK FISH

FOOD	PORTION	CAL	PRO	VIT C	FOL	CA	IR
raw	3½ oz	79	17	–	tr	17	–

FOOD	PORTION	CAL	PRO	VIT C	FOL	CA	IR
VEAL							
FRESH							
cubed, lean only, raw	1 oz	31	6	–	4	5	tr
cutlet, lean only; braised	3 oz	172	31	–	15	7	1
cutlet, lean only; fried	3 oz	156	28	–	14	6	1
ground, raw	1 oz	41	5	–	4	4	tr
ground; broiled	3 oz	146	21	–	10	14	1
loin chop w/ bone, lean & fat, raw	1 chop (4.4 oz)	204	24	–	17	20	1
loin chop w/ bone, lean & fat; braised	1 chop (2.8 oz)	227	24	–	11	22	1
loin chop w/ bone, lean only; braised	1 chop (2.4 oz)	155	23	–	10	22	1
shoulder w/ bone, lean only, braised	3 oz	169	29	–	14	31	1
sirloin w/ bone, lean & fat; roasted	3 oz	171	21	–	13	11	1
sirloin w/ bone, lean only; roasted	3 oz	143	22	–	13	12	1
VEGETABLES MIXED							
CANNED							
mixed vegetables	½ cup	39	2	4	19	22	1
peas & carrots	½ cup	48	3	8	24	29	1
peas & onions	½ cup	30	2	2	–	10	1
succotash	½ cup	102	4	9	59	15	1
FROZEN							
mixed vegetables; cooked	½ cup	54	3	3	17	22	1
peas & carrots; cooked	½ cup	38	3	7	21	18	1
peas & onions; cooked	½ cup	40	2	6	–	13	1
succotash; cooked	½ cup	79	4	5	28	13	1
HOME RECIPE							
succotash	½ cup	111	5	8	–	16	1

FOOD	PORTION	CAL	PRO	VIT C	FOL	CA	IR
JUICE							
vegetable juice cocktail	6 oz	34	1	50	–	20	1
vegetable juice cocktail	½ cup	22	1	34	–	13	1
VENISON							
raw	1 oz	34	7	–	–	1	1
roasted	3 oz	134	26	–	–	6	4
VINEGAR							
cider	1 tbsp	tr	tr	0	–	1	tr
WAFFLES							
HOME RECIPE							
waffle	7" diam	245	7	tr	–	154	2
MIX							
as prep w/ egg & milk	1 waffle (2.6 oz)	205	7	tr	–	179	1
WALNUTS							
black, dried	1 oz	172	7	–	–	16	1
black, dried; chopped	1 cup	759	30	–	–	72	4
english, dried	1 oz	182	4	1	19	27	1
english, dried; chopped	1 cup	770	17	4	79	113	3
WATER CHESTNUTS							
CANNED							
chinese, salted	½ cup	35	1	1	–	3	1
FRESH							
sliced	½ cup	66	1	3	–	7	tr
WATERCRESS							
raw; chopped	½ cup	2	tr	7	–	20	t
WATERMELON							
cut up	1 cup	50	1	15	3	13	t

FOOD	PORTION	CAL	PRO	VIT C	FOL	CA	IR
wedge	1/16	152	3	47	10	38	1
SEEDS							
dried	1 oz	158	8	–	16	15	2
dried	1 cup	602	8	0	16	15	2

WHALE

raw	3.5 oz	134	23	–	–	12	4

WHEAT

sprouted	1/3 cup	71	3	tr	–	10	tr
starch	3½ oz	348	tr	0	–	0	0

WHEAT GERM

toasted	1/4 cup	108	8	2	100	13	3
untoasted	1/4 cup	104	7	0	82	11	2

WHELK (SNAIL)

FRESH							
cooked	3 oz	233	41	–	10	96	9
raw	3 oz	117	20	–	5	48	4

WHIPPED TOPPINGS

cream, pressurized	1 tbsp	8	tr	0	–	3	tr
cream, pressurized	1 cup	154	2	0	–	61	tr
nondairy, powdered; as prep w/ whole milk	1 tbsp	8	tr	tr	tr	4	tr
nondairy, powdered; as prep w/ whole milk	1 cup	151	3	1	3	72	tr
nondairy, pressurized	1 tbsp	11	tr	0	0	tr	tr
nondairy, pressurized	1 cup	184	1	0	0	4	tr
nondairy, frzn	1 tbsp	13	tr	0	0	tr	tr

FOOD	PORTION	CAL	PRO	VIT C	FOL	CA	IR
WHITE BEANS							
CANNED							
white beans	1 cup	306	19	0	171	191	8
DRIED							
regular, raw	1 cup	674	47	0	783	486	21
regular; cooked	1 cup	249	17	0	145	161	7
small, raw	1 cup	723	45	0	830	373	17
small; cooked	1 cup	253	16	0	245	131	5
WHITEFISH							
FRESH							
raw	3 oz	114	16	–	–	–	tr
SMOKED							
whitefish	1 oz	39	7	–	2	5	tr
whitefish	3 oz	92	20	–	6	15	tr
WHITING							
FRESH							
cooked	3 oz	98	20	–	13	53	tr
raw	3 oz	77	16	–	11	41	tr
WILD RICE							
cooked	½ cup	83	3	0	22	3	tr
raw	½ cup	286	12	0	76	17	2
WINE							
red	3½ oz	74	tr	0	2	8	tr
rose	3½ oz	73	tr	0	1	9	tr
sweet dessert	2 oz	90	tr	0	tr	5	tr
white	3½ oz	70	tr	0	tr	9	tr

FOOD	PORTION	CAL	PRO	VIT C	FOL	CA	IR
WINGED BEANS							
DRIED							
cooked	1 cup	252	18	0	18	244	7
raw	1 cup	745	54	0	81	800	24
WOLFFISH							
FRESH							
atlantic, raw	3 oz	82	15	–	–	–	tr
YAM							
mountain yam, hawaii; cooked	½ cup	59	1	0	–	6	tr
yam; cubed, cooked	½ cup	79	1	8	11	9	tr
YARDLONG BEANS							
DRIED							
cooked	1 cup	202	14	1	249	72	5
raw	1 cup	580	41	3	1099	230	14
YEAST							
baker's dry active	1 pkg (7 g)	20	3	tr	–	3	1
brewer's dry	1 tbsp	25	3	tr	–	17	1
YELLOW BEANS							
DRIED							
cooked	1 cup	254	16	3	143	110	4
raw	1 cup	676	43	0	762	325	14
YELLOWTAIL							
FRESH							
raw	3 oz	124	20	2	3	–	tr
YOGURT							
coffee, lowfat	8 oz	194	11	2	24	389	tr
fruit, lowfat	4 oz	113	5	1	10	157	tr

FOOD	PORTION	CAL	PRO	VIT C	FOL	CA	IR
fruit, lowfat	8 oz	225	9	1	19	314	tr
plain	8 oz	139	8	1	17	274	tr
plain, lowfat	8 oz	144	12	2	25	415	tr
plain, no fat	8 oz	127	13	2	28	452	tr
vanilla, lowfat	8 oz	194	11	2	24	389	tr

ZUCCHINI

FOOD	PORTION	CAL	PRO	VIT C	FOL	CA	IR
CANNED							
italian style	½ cup	33	1	3	–	19	1
FRESH							
raw; sliced	½ cup	9	1	6	14	10	tr
sliced, cooked	½ cup	14	1	4	15	12	tr
FROZEN							
cooked	½ cup	19	1	4	9	19	1

Index

T = Table